Strong Shadows

Scenes from an Inner City AIDS Clinic

Strong Shadows

Scenes from an Inner City AIDS Clinic

Abigail Zuger, M.D.

There is strong shadow where there is much light.
—Goethe

The chapter on Shannon Gallagher was first published in a different form in *Discover* magazine, July 1993.

The chapter on Nancy Corelli first appeared in *The New York Times Magazine*, July 25, 1993.

Library of Congress Cataloging-in-Publication Data

Zuger, Abigail.
    Strong shadows : scenes from an inner city AIDS clinic/
Abigail Zuger.
        p.   cm.
    ISBN 0-7167-2916-4
    1. AIDS (Disease)—Case studies.   2. Poor—
Medical care—Case studies.   3. Inner cities.   I. Title.
    RC607.A26Z84   1995
    362.1'969792—dc20   95-7587
                                                        CIP

Printed in the United States of America

First printing 1995, VB

For B. Z. and M. T. Z.—
my anchor and my sails

Contents

Preface

Everyone has had an introduction to AIDS. Mine came during the first month of my medical internship at Bellevue Hospital in New York City. It was early dawn on a July day in 1981, and the second-year resident anxiously supervising my every nighttime move still wouldn't let me go lie down. Instead, I was to go back to the bedside of a man I had just admitted with pneumonia, wake him up, and ask him *why* he wasn't married.

I told Chris she was crazy. If ever a question could wait until morning, not to say forever, this was the one. She knew otherwise. "Look," she snapped, "there's something going around . . . Oh, forget it. It's too complicated. I'll go talk to him myself."

Chris knew what I was soon to learn. The fledgling disease without a name—the Centers for Disease Control had formally acknowledged its existence only a month before—was everywhere in New York's public hospitals. Over the next few years I too would confront with amazement and frustration the chasm that separated our reality in the hospital from the rest of the world's. In the early 1980s our wards were full of patients with a disease almost no one else could imagine. "There's something going around," I would begin. "Oh, forget it." It was too complicated, too unbelievable, to explain.

Those days, of course, are over; everybody wears the red ribbon now. AIDS is long out of the closet, with spokespersons and foundations, million-dollar budgets, a commision and a czar. AZT and vaccine trials are dinner-table conversation. Novels and movies, sitcoms and confessionals, have all presented to the American public one face of AIDS.

Other faces remain in the background, shadowed but no less real. While the impact of HIV on the gay community is well described, the panorama of HIV infection among the urban poor, a world in which I still work, remains utterly unfamiliar to the rest of our society. The intersecting crises of illicit drug use, poverty, and terminal disease may get their bites in the daily news, but nothing I've read or seen does justice to the steady drizzle of human loss HIV has brought to the inner city. The media focus on the crises; the crowd of faces caught within the crises stays blank.

I wrote this book to fill in the faces, to give them mouths and let them speak. Our patients are far more eloquent historians of their times and their disease than media reporters and salaried spokespersons alike. I didn't want their part of the history of AIDS to be forgotten.

Middle-class Americans will have difficulty recognizing the background of misery and chaos against which our patients cope with their miserable, chaotic disease. Drug use and sexual contact have sent the virus into every corner of their universe. They are as likely as not to be the fourth or fifth or tenth member of their circle of family and friends to be infected, sharing diagnoses and doctors with parents, siblings, spouses, and children. Medical crises are juggled with dozens of others: court dates and parole violations, fostered-out children and strung-out parents, vandalized apartments, errant bullets, empty refrigerators, disconnected phones. The medications we judiciously prescribe are as likely as not to be sold on the corner for the price of a week's groceries or bartered for "better pills, you know, the ones my brother gets," or for a bag of dope. The No. 4 subway train may serve for their final ambulance, and their cortege.

But HIV derails hopes and promise no less efficiently in this world than it does anywhere else. "I didn't mean for it to be like this," they say. "I was just a kid back then. I've been off the stuff for six years now"—or for ten years, or for a dozen—off the streets, in a program, back in school, in a good job, haven't seen that man in years, just got married, just had a fine fat little baby, just slipped up once, or twice, or not at all, just was planning to pick up the pieces, and now this. "Help me fight this thing," they ask us, no different from anyone else. "I don't deserve this. How can this be happening to me?"

Ideally, I would have liked to mount a camera in a corner of my examining room, point it at the chair next to my desk where the patient sits, and let it run. Failing this option, I have tried to achieve the same result with words. I have changed names and some details to protect the identities of patients and their families, but otherwise, this is a documentary book.

Readers will find that AIDS in the inner city has less to do with sexual politics than with individual citizenship, less with abstractions of art and mortality than with the mundanities of food, shelter, child care, and Medicaid cards. No disease shows up the crazy quilt of American medical care for the shabby thing it is among the sick-to-death poor better than AIDS. In the infectious disease clinics of large urban hospitals like mine, the much-touted amenities of our health-care system are not in evidence. Patients often wait half a day for a fifteen-minute appointment during a jammed first-come, first-served clinic session. Far from choosing their own doctor, they become inured to doctors fading unpredictably in and out of their lives, while battalions of doctors-in-training march on through. State-of-the-art medical innovations—same-day surgery, home intravenous antibiotics—are generally unavailable. All off-hours care takes place in a frantic, blood-spattered emergency room. When patients are admitted into the hospital, the doctor legally responsible for their care is usually one they've never met.

These features of urban health care are not intended cruelties; they are simply the form into which "poverty medicine" has evolved in our for-profit system. At some point in the future, nationally legislated health-care reform may erase them all. Meanwhile, paradoxically, some of the best AIDS medicine in the country is practiced in these shabby urban HIV clinics—testament to the degree to which the energy, insight, and compassion of hospital staff can offset the worst administrative shortsightedness and neglect.

This book tells the stories of a few of the dozens of patients who took their places on the chair opposite my clinic desk during the early 1990s, at the beginning of the second decade of AIDS. In the 1980s the medical care we could provide for patients like them was primeval; in the 1990s it has evolved to the merely primitive. Thanks to a decade of furious research we have a few basic treatment tools: a test for HIV, a few toxic and not very effective drugs for controlling it, a sense of the natural history of HIV and of the infections and tumors it causes, and some techniques for treating and preventing them. Optimism dictates that, like the clinic described in this book, the diseases and treatments discussed will soon also be obsolete. Sadly, as of this writing, virtually none of them is.

These stories are focused on our patients and their families. We who work in the clinic, ripe though we too may be for analysis, are purposely kept to the background. Some parts of our own stories—what keeps some of us at this kind of job and drives some of us away—will come through nonetheless, for AIDS has brought a whole new chapter to the social history of medical care and caretakers. But that chapter is, by rights, part of another book. For this book, our patients have the stage.

I am an internist and infectious disease specialist, as are most of the doctors with whom I work. The infectious disease clinic suite, where I spent an afternoon a week during the years spanned by this book, is located in the hospital's outpatient building. A door off the main fourth-floor corridor opens into a large waiting room, with a reception counter by the entrance and a tangle of overgrown plants by a large bay window opposite. Thirty or forty patients can fit into the waiting room, sitting on an assortment of battered couches and interlocking hard plastic chairs. Off either end of the waiting room two narrow corridors lead to a total of nine small consultation rooms. On a busy day, with twenty-five or thirty patients to be seen, five doctors, two or three nurses, a social worker, and a nutritionist share these rooms. The social worker occasionally makes do on a couch in the corridor outside. Each consultation room contains a few chairs and a desk. Most have examining tables and telephones. Some, prime real estate, have sinks. For my Wednesday sessions, I try very hard always to snag a room with a sink.

Patients come into the clinic, check in with the receptionist behind the counter, have a seat in the waiting room, and wait. They are called into a side room by a nurse, interviewed, have their temperature and blood pressure taken, have a seat in the waiting room again, and wait. Their charts are placed in a wooden box on the door of the doctor's cubicle. During the minutes or hours patients wait for their doctor—we try, not always successfully, to have them see the same doctor at every visit—they have time to see the nutritionist or social worker if they choose. When patients are finished with all their appointments, they have a seat in the waiting room once more and wait. They are called by a nurse to review the doctor's instructions and then return to the reception counter, where the receptionist gives them follow-up appointments and X-ray or blood-test slips to present at the lab. Then they are sent on their way.

I seldom see more than half a dozen patients in the course of a Wednesday afternoon—not very many by most standards, but these patients are sick and complicated, the paperwork for each visit is extensive, and the whole process takes time. I go in order of arrival, working my way through the stack of charts in the box on my door. I pick up the chart, leaf through it to refresh my memory of the patient, walk the short length of corridor into the waiting room, call the patient's name, and the visit begins.

Deborah Sweet

JULY 1991

Deborah Sweet is balanced on the little chair by my desk, leaning forward and looking deep into my eyes. One of my hands is clasped firmly between both of hers. "I'm real, *real* glad you're gonna be my doctor," she says. "I know we're gonna get along just fine."

I wish I could say the same, but Deborah has been raising hell in the clinic for two years now and I know we're not gonna get along at all. No one ever gets along with Deborah. She is handed from doctor to doctor like a sputtering grenade. Last month the clinic director decided that perhaps a firm and experienced hand like mine was what Deborah really needed, and hence her dog-eared chart is now sitting on my desk and Deborah is sitting on my examining room chair, slathering me with loving-kindness.

She is a tall, heavy, middle-aged woman with dyed orange hair. One of her big gold earrings is ripping through an earlobe. The leather handbag on her lap is overflowing: I glimpse a Bible, an empty pill bottle, and a handful of tattered envelopes that undoubtedly contain forms for me to fill out. But Deborah is too savvy to get to the forms right away. She knows that first impressions are important.

Unfortunately, I've learned a good deal about Deborah already. The aunt who raised her since she was orphaned as an infant is a nurse who used to work at our hospital. Many of our clinic nurses are good friends of the family, although too loyal to comment directly on Deborah's career save with a shake of the head. A smart girl from a solid background, she apparently was given every advantage and went straight to hell. From what I have pieced together, nothing more exotic was involved than a lot of drugs, a little prostitution, and a smidgen of petty theft. In between, Deborah finished a few semesters of college and married several times, most recently to a Mr. White. She, her husband, her aunt and her uncle, reunited now by the compromises of illness, poverty, and old age, share a two-family house near the hospital. Her two grown children live in another state.

I am considerably more familiar with Deborah's clinic career than with her private life, since her voice tends to penetrate doors and walls. She was diagnosed with AIDS during a hospital admission for pneumonia in 1989. The doctor who took care of her during that admission was an old professional friend of her aunt's, one of the neighborhood's more genteel private practitioners. After Deborah's discharge he suggested that she should come to our clinic for her follow-up care, since his familiarity with the medications used to treat HIV infection was limited. Was this ground for transfer coincidence or prescience on his part? How did he know that medications are precisely the cause of so many hard feelings between Deb and her physicians? She is still behaving beautifully in Dr. Schwartz's office when her aunt brings her in to him for intermittent checkups. Her tantrums are reserved for us.

Deborah has had no further episodes of pneumonia or other infections since her AIDS diagnosis. Rather, her ongoing medical problems all predate this most recent assault on her health. She has chronic anxiety for which she takes Ativan (a sedative related to Valium, 1 milligram three times daily). She has chronic hip pain from a long-ago car accident, for which she takes Darvocet (100 milligrams three times daily). She has a history of seizures from an old concussion, for which she takes Dilantin (100 milligrams three times daily) and phenobarbital (30 milligrams four times daily). She has a peptic ulcer, for which she needs Zantac, and an asthmatic condition, for which she needs a Ventolin inhaler. And, of course, she takes AZT to slow the progress of her HIV infection.

So far, no problem. This has been the problem: "Excuse me, Doctor, but you did not. You most certainly did not give me my Ativan last time. You said you were going to but you did not. I got home and I didn't have the prescription. I didn't have it anywhere. And I need my medicine. That's what I've come back for. I don't care what you wrote in that chart. YOU DIDN'T GIVE IT TO ME. I DON'T CARE WHAT YOU SAY. YOU GIVE IT TO ME NOW. YOU GIVE IT TO ME NOW OR I'LL DO SOMETHING TO YOU. YES I WILL, RIGHT IN YOUR WHITE FACE. YOU TREAT ALL BLACK PEOPLE THIS WAY, DOCTOR?" And once she is off, nothing works to stop her, neither soft words nor security guards, nothing but the prescription for whatever it was, which was mysteriously absent from her medications at her last visit, or which she lost in a fight at Yankee Stadium yesterday, or which was stolen from her car, or which was taken out of her handbag on the train. When the desired prescription is safe in hand she strides out, vowing under her breath never to return. But she always does.

We figure Deborah is as good as a ticker tape for monitoring the street value of prescription drugs. Ativan is hot one week, Darvocet the next; Zantac and Ventolin, both said to potentiate a cocaine high, are always in demand. AZT is a new addition to the street pharmacopoeia but gaining in popularity. She is probably taking next to none of the medication herself: she certainly has a lot of vigor to be ingesting much Ativan, and her blood Dilantin levels—routinely used to monitor therapy—have usually been negative. The changes AZT causes in the shape and size of the red blood cells are nowhere to be found in Deborah's blood smears.

Not that many of Deborah's blood smears are to be found either. In fact, when I looked through her chart before calling her into the room, I couldn't find any blood results less than two years old. Ordinarily we order blood tests at least every few months for someone taking AZT. But of course, Deborah probably isn't taking AZT, and the day she was confronted with this hypothesis was, I imagine, the day she decided she might as well stop getting her blood drawn. She has the arms of a hard-core drug injector—scarred and thick-skinned, all the superficial veins dissolved long ago. Obtaining blood from arms like hers requires patience, skill, and a considerable time commitment, while the easier and less painful alternative of puncturing the big vessels in her neck or groin mandates her assent and cooperation. None of these commodities is in particular evidence in her chart, and no blood results either. What to do?

What to do but to look back deeply into Deborah's eyes and smile hard. First impressions are, after all, important.

"I'm very glad to be taking care of you, Ms. Sweet."

She releases my hand and leans back, satisfied.

"I've just been looking through your chart here to get to know you a little. It looks to me like you've been feeling pretty well."

It certainly does. For someone who has had AIDS for three years, Deborah looks like a million dollars. She is hefty and sleek, her skin clear, her voice strong as she leans back in the chair and says smugly, "Well, now, that's because I take my medication, Doctor, especially my A-to-Z."

Her A-to-Z? Her AZT.

"How much of that AZT are you taking these days, Ms. Sweet?"

"I take 200 milligrams every four hours, five times per day, Doctor. That doctor before you tried to cut me down, but I told him no, that's my dose that I take and that's the dose that's keeping me well, and that's the dose I take, is all. He was no good, anyhow."

She is completely accurate. Deborah's last clinic visit did in fact terminate, loudly, with her insistence on obtaining prescriptions for an outdated AZT dosage, twice as much as has been used in patients for several years. I feel a little bolder, remembering this. She has never staged two scenes in a row. I look her in the eye.

"That's too much AZT for a lady who doesn't get blood tests."

"You think I look sick, Doctor?" The smile is gone from her face and she sounds fierce.

"That dose of AZT can do a lot of damage to a person's red blood cells without showing up in how they look."

"What you driving at, Doctor?"

"I want to keep you as healthy as possible, Ms. Sweet. That's why I'm not going to give you any more AZT until I see how your blood count's doing." A bold stroke. I hold my breath, but Deborah is unfazed.

"I get my blood tests, Doctor. My doctor, Dr. Schwartz, does my blood tests. I just come here for my medicines."

The thought of the elderly, elegant Dr. Schwartz, his nurse, or any laboratory he does business with dealing with Deborah's arms, neck, or groin is comical. Only hospital hacks with years of ongoing experience drawing blood from drug users (or drug users themselves) can successfully tap extremities like hers.

"Well, I'm sure Dr. Schwartz fills out your blood slips for you. But I bet they have a hard time in his lab with those arms of yours."

Silence.

"And then I bet they send you back to his office so he can draw your blood himself."

Silence.

"And then I bet you don't go."

Silence.

"And then I bet you tell him that we're checking your blood here so he doesn't have to bother."

Silence.

"You know, I can take blood from your groin in three seconds and it won't even hurt."

She looks dubious.

"And then I get my A-to-Z?"

I look dubious.

But this is how, ten minutes later, I have two warm tubes of blood labeled and safely swathed in plastic on my desk and Deborah Sweet has a prescription for an obsolete and dangerous dose of AZT in her fist.

"You see, Doctor," she says as she reaches into her purse for the SSI (Supplemental Security Income)/ disability and housing forms I have to fill out and sign. "I told you we were going to get along real well. Don't forget to write me for my Ativan today."

July 1991

February 1992

Mary, the head nurse in the clinic, rolls her eyes as she puts Deborah Sweet's chart in my box but doesn't say a word. This is worrisome, although difficult to interpret. Anything could be going on. In the eight months that I have been taking care of Deborah I have seen her seven times, and each visit has been a carefully orchestrated choreography of wills, of small concessions to serve bigger aims that leaves me exhausted. I have scored several victories of principle: Deborah now accepts prescriptions

for a standard dose of AZT, as well as for her other medications, at regular monthly intervals. We count the slips
out together, and the return visits for lost prescriptions
have stopped. Every month I tap her groin for a few tubes
of blood.

Over the course of our acquaintance, Deborah has
slowly caught up on most of her routine screening blood
tests, including her syphilis serology (negative), her
hepatitis serology (positive), and her T-helper-cell count
(disturbingly low at 19). The white blood cell called the
T-helper cell is one of HIV's major targets for destruction,
and the number of these cells that have disappeared from
the circulation correlates fairly well with an infected person's degree of immunosuppression. If their T-helper-cell
counts are in the normal 500 to 1,000 range, most HIV-
infected people fight off infection quite well. The further
their counts fall below 100 to 200, the more vulnerable to
infection they become. I looked at Deborah's T-cell
results for a long time when they showed up in my box.
The process of coping with the vigorous, powerful, endlessly resourceful Deborah tended to move the real reason for our acquaintance to the very back of my mind,
but here was an inescapable reminder.

When I told Deborah about her T-cell count last
month, she hadn't seemed very interested. Her agenda
for that visit were the itchy, infected pustules on the back
of an ear she had just had repierced and the bruises over
her right cheek left over from a recent mugging. She also
had a few choice words to say about a psychiatrist to

whom I had referred her the month before. She had begun to lobby for an increase in her Ativan dose, and I smelled trouble ahead. I hated the thought of antagonizing my new peaceful, palliated Deborah, and I had hoped that a psychiatrist experienced in drug-seeking behavior might make a few suggestions, might even take an intellectual interest in her idiosyncratic blend of personality disorders and see her regularly, might conceivably even take over the job of writing her tranquilizer prescriptions.

No such luck. Dr. Burton and Deborah did not get along. "I'm not going back there," she stated flatly. "He told me I take drugs. I don't take drugs, not in years. Any anyway, he said he's in trouble with the law. No way I'm getting mixed up with him. I stay out of trouble."

Dr. Burton, when I reached him later on the phone, had clarified somewhat. "I told her I don't prescribe Ativan. A patient stole one of my prescription pads last year and forged my name to forty Ativan prescriptions. It took a while to straighten it out." He paused. "Actually, I think it's really malpractice to give these patients Ativan. I tell them that straight out. They only sell it. You should think about what you're doing." Accurate though this might be, it was not helpful. At the end of the conversation, I tended to share Deborah's opinion of Dr. Burton.

In comparison with an oozing, crusted ear, a bruised and aching cheekbone, and the deflating experience of Dr. Burton, Deborah's T-cell count had seemed barely to register last month, and I hadn't particularly wanted to alarm her by dwelling on it. Now, glancing at her vital signs on today's clinic sheet before I call her into my room, I remember her results anew. On paper, at least, it looks like Deborah is dying.

"Patient is extremely weak with unsteady gait," says the nursing assessment. "Has no appetite. Weight down 7 lbs. Night sweats. No cough. Blood pressure could not be obtained. Temp 98.2°. Pulse thready."

It's not hard to find Deborah in the crowded waiting room. She's slumped over on the couch, head in the lap of a middle-aged man I've never seen before. A wheelchair is parked next to them, blocking the seats on the rest of the couch and forming a small clearing for their tableau. "Deborah?" I say. She barely moves. Her companion looks at me and shakes his head, exactly the way Mary had a few minutes before. "Mr. White," he says. "Deb's husband." Between us, we load her into the wheelchair and back to the examining room. From the banks of hard chairs across from the couch, the other waiting patients watch us impassively.

In the examining room Deborah's husband proves to be a man of few words. "She ain't feeling too good," he says.

"It's my ulcer," Deborah murmurs through cracked lips. "My ulcer is acting up again."

"She ain't eaten nothing in one, two weeks," supplies her husband.

"It hurts when I eat," moans Deborah. "I try to take in fluids like my aunt says but I can't." She begins to slip out of the wheelchair like a rag doll. "Can I lie down for a minute?" she asks.

Hoisting her dead weight up onto the examining table winds all of us. Mr. White excuses himself to recover outside, while Deborah lies splayed on the table and I, my concern seasoned with more than a little guilt (How could I have begrudged Deborah that Zantac? How miserably hard and suspicious I am becoming!), set about checking her out for blood loss and dehydration, two major sequelae of an active ulcer.

Deborah checks out just fine. Her unobtainable blood pressure turns out to be quite normal, the usual sounds simply muffled by the thick scars in her forearms. The pulse at her wrist is slow, strong, regular. Her abdomen is soft. A pelvic exam is normal. She has no evidence of internal bleeding. A rapid check on her red blood cell count shows it is unchanged from its usual value. She has a few small white patches of the candida infection called thrush in her mouth, as she has had occasionally in the past. That's it.

By the time I've come back from running her blood up to the lab, Deborah has made herself more comfortable on the examining table. She is reclining on her right side, facing the room, right hand supporting her head, left hand resting casually on her left hip. It occurs to me that she looks a little like Elizabeth Taylor as Cleopatra, pre-asp. Armed with data, I've stopped feeling guilty.

"Deborah, everything's checking out OK. How are you feeling?"

"I feel terrible, Dr. Zuger, just terrible. I can't eat."

"You have a little thrush in your mouth. You've had that before. It may have moved down your throat a little. Maybe that's why you can't eat."

"Maybe so, Dr. Zuger. Maybe so."

"I'm going to give you a pill that should clear that up in a few days. Do you think you can get a pill down?"

"I'll try, Dr. Zuger. I'll surely try."

"I don't think it's your ulcer, Deborah."

"Maybe not, Dr. Zuger. Maybe not." She rolls herself to a sitting position, still a little gray but pretty steady.

Something is definitely up here. What in the world can it be? I had figured it was a run on the Zantac market, but Deborah appears completely content to quit the lists today with Diflucan, a medication for thrush, not Zantac, dangling from her lance. Has Diflucan got itself a market value? A definite possibility—it's certainly a handy drug to have on hand. Alternatively (What is the matter with me? Have I learned no humility from the preceding half hour?), maybe Deborah does in fact have a candida infection in her esophagus, a white coating of yeast snaking down her throat, leaving it raw and inflamed, making swallowing painful and difficult. This condition is so common in AIDS patients that we generally don't even bother ordering confirmatory X rays of the esophagus. We treat for it presumptively, and if the patients get better, that's what they had.

But if this is the case, then why is Deborah starting to recover before my very eyes? Maybe the usual routine of the examining room—the letting of blood, the laying on of hands—has in fact soothed her, quieted her pain, steadied her as these therapeutics did in the Middle Ages. . . . I will try to remember that this is a patient here. A sick, terminal patient, not an opponent in the lists.

"OK, Deborah, this is a prescription for Diflucan I'm going to give to your husband. He should get it filled right away. I want you to take two today, then one every morning. And I want you to come back next week so we can see how you're doing. I'm worried about you, Deborah!"

She nods quietly and lets herself be helped into the wheelchair. I wheel her back out into the examining room and deliver her to her husband, now sitting majestically alone on the couch. He nods when I tell him about the fungus and pockets the prescription. Deborah leans over, tugs on his jacket, whispers in his ear. To my surprise, when I head back to the examining room, Mr. White is behind me.

"Dr. Zuger, Deborah, she just remember, she got a court date coming up tomorrow. They say she gotta show up or get a letter from you saying she's too sick to go to court."

I write a short note to whom it may concern. Deborah Sweet is under my ongoing care for . . . for what? For acute distress? For symptoms without signs? For major inability to attend court sessions? For immune problems with periodic exacerbations. For what ails her. I knew something was up. When I deliver the note to Mr. White, Deborah is standing up, briskly folding up the wheelchair in preparation for departure. "I feel so much better after talking to you, Doctor," she explains.

July 1991
February 1992
....
August 1992
....

When I get to the clinic this afternoon, the waiting room is sunny and blissfully silent. Two nurses are chatting softly behind the reception desk, and a solitary patient, face half-masked by a stocking cap, snoozes in a corner chair. But as I work my way through the stack of mail waiting on my desk, a vague, unfamiliar murmur coming from the waiting room begins to itch my concentration away from blood-test results, prescription renewals, and visiting nurse reports. It's nothing I can place immediately, none of the usual attention shatterers, not the penetrating crystal-cracking inflections of Simone, the Jamaican nurse, discussing her little girl's braces, nor the muted wheedle of a patient at the desk trying to convince Mary he needs to be seen today. It's too early for the sound of Oprah or any of the others to be emanating from the TV suspended in one corner of the waiting room, although this murmur has that same endless whiny rise and fall as a muffled television, that same persistent rhythm, that same nagging demand to be heard. I realize I am now reading the report of Angel Candelario's visiting nurse for the fifth time.

Mary skids by my door, deposits a chart in my box, vanishes. "Hey," I call after her. "Hey, what is going on out there?" No answer, she hasn't heard me. But that strange noise is continuing, a muted tune, almost a song, a plain-song, now merging into a background of the usual clinic session noises, phones ringing, patients talking, children crying, nurses summoning. There's no alternative to getting up and seeing what's going on for myself. As I get to the door of my room Mary glides up from the other direction. She bares her teeth in a cheerless grin. "Don't ask," she says.

If I walk out of my examining room and a few steps to the right I can look into the waiting room without being too noticeable myself. A good crowd of patients has showed up by now, camped over the rows of interlocking plastic chairs with relatives, attendants, strollers. Some are still chomping on lunches of hot dogs with sauerkraut and onions—the Sabrett vendor at the building entrance does a brisk business with the afternoon clinic crowd. In the middle of the waiting room a small clearing has formed around a disheveled figure who, sitting on a bank of plastic chairs and wildly waving a hot-dog stub, is energetically preaching to the crowd.

This is what I've been hearing, muted by corners and a corridor. Now the chant is all too clear. "Hallelujah, I do know I will be saved," announces Deborah, eyes closed and arms embracing the room. "I have sinned and I have this virus that is my sin, but Jesus Christ has forgiven me, and I will be saved from this virus!" A few tentative "amens" follow this declaration. Deborah opens her eyes and looks right at me. "I will be saved!" she announces, rising, pointing her hot dog at me. "I *will* be saved!"

Twenty pairs of eyes follow the pointer of Deborah's hot dog to me in my alcove. This is a cue in a million; for one moment I am tempted to throw discretion to the winds and march into the waiting room hollering "Amen!"—arms outstretched toward Deborah's hot dog, white coat floating behind me, a healer incarnate. Instead, I hastily slink back several paces out of sight. In the waiting room all is quiet. Then Deborah's voice appears again, no longer chanting but quite loud and matter-of-fact. "She hates black folks," I hear her say to no one in particular. "They all do."

Deborah made an astounding recovery from her brush with whatever it was last winter. One week later she strode purposefully into the clinic pushing her handbag in the wheelchair, six pounds heavier, not a complaint in the world. Diflucan can accomplish these miracles some-times, and so, of course, can rescheduled court dates. I am consciously trying to avoid deciding which was respon-sible for the miracle here. I have kept Deborah supplied with Diflucan and reassured the assistant district attorney who called to inquire about her health that ups and downs are typical of her disease process. The state alleges that Deborah held up a taxicab several years ago, but the ADA, young and kindly on the other end of the phone, was only wondering if he shouldn't drop all charges in view of her terminal condition.

Had he been wandering through the waiting room today, he might have reconsidered his instincts toward clemency. The hot dog has vanished, but Deborah has risen, eyes closed, and is swaying back and forth, crooning. She has lost some of her audience—a small relocation out of the waiting room into the main corridor has taken place—but of the remaining patients, a few seem actually to be swaying slightly in place beside her. Mary, on the other hand, standing behind me outside my examining room, has gone quite rigid. "Now what?" she asks.

We have never really perfected a system for dealing with the occasional psychotic break we host in the clinic, let alone for what promises to develop into a full-fledged tent meeting. It is only at moments like this that the deficiency really hits home. In theory, our procedure is the same as the rest of the hospital's: acutely psychotic, violent, threatening, or suicidal patients are to be escorted by a doctor and a security guard down to the emergency room, where the staff is trained and prepared to cope with this kind of behavior. In fact, we can never accomplish the transfer with any kind of finesse. Our patients know and hate the emergency room, and the less rational they are, the deeper and more visceral their hatred seems to become. When they hear the words "emergency room" they invariably flee, sometimes unchallenged, sometimes pursued by a security guard who never seems to pursue too fast.

When fleeing patients are violent, threatening, or weapon-bearing, we are not unhappy to watch them scamper down the corridor toward other venues. But when they are suicidally depressed or temporarily delirious for some medical reason, we realize all over again that we badly need some constructive scheme for handling them. Toward this end, we have been cultivating a collaboration with the group of psychiatrists in the hospital who have a professional interest in the psychiatry of HIV infection and a large cash grant from the government to study it. We agreed a few months ago that one of the psychiatrists would be our backup during each clinic session and would, if the circumstances justified it, make the two-block trek from their offices to the clinic to help with the emergency.

And what better time to call for our backup than now?

"Hi, Dan?" Unfortunately, the backup of the day is Dr. Burton, whose mettle Deborah and I both had assayed and found wanting several months previously. But at least he knows her case.

"Dan, we have a little situation here that we're not really sure how to deal with . . ."

Dr. Burton is unimpressed by the evangelical details.

"She has to go to the emergency room."

"Look, Dan, she won't go. I know she won't. She's praying and she's paranoid. She'll just head out the door. I think this situation really needs someone with experience. A security guard would just make things worse. We'd really appreciate it if you gave us a hand." Always appeal to kindness, however latent it may appear to be.

But Dr. Burton is implacable. "I'm really tied up right now. I told you she shouldn't be getting Ativan. She's probably going to tell you she's withdrawing. Wants a higher dose now. I told you it was trouble. They'll calm her down in the ER."

"Dan, we're having a revival meeting here. What do I do about it?"

"Good luck." And he's gone. Mary leans against the door and looks grim. "Well, I'm not calling Security," she says. "Absolutely not. And you're not either. It would turn into a riot."

The alternatives seem to be dwindling rapidly down to one. I pick Deborah's chart out of the box on my door and head out to the waiting room. "Ms. Sweet?"

Deborah stops mid-croon, gathers up her purse and sweater, pauses to throw her onion-stained paper napkin into the wastebasket, and, head high, precedes me out of the waiting room. Behind us I hear the stirrings of hidden patients resuming their seats. The nurses begin to murmur. Deborah sits down in the examining room chair, feet planted firmly on the floor, and stares at me as I carefully leave the door open a few inches and lean on the examining table opposite her. Were I to sit in my usual seat, she would be between me and the door. I paste a calm smile on my face.

"How are you, Deborah?"

"I have wax in my ears and a urine infection. And how come you're not doing anything about it?"

"I'm sorry, Deborah, I didn't know about either of those. Do you have pain when you pass your urine?"

"No, I don't." Her stare intensifies. I can see the whites of her eyes.

"Do you have fever or pain in your belly?"

"No, I don't."

"Then how—"

"They took urine at my program and said I couldn't come back because I had an infection. THAT'S HOW COME. SO YOU BETTER DO SOMETHING, DOCTOR, BECAUSE BLACK PEOPLE DON'T GET NO CARE AROUND HERE AND THAT'S A FACT."

I have been hearing Deborah intermittently through the walls during the last three years, and this free-form surfboarding across waves of thought is typical of her worst days. Still, I would be remiss not to at least consider the possibility that, as with any of our patients who begin to behave strangely, she has finally succumbed to one of the AIDS-related brain conditions that show up as paranoia or a thought disorder and can potentially be cured. As much as I hate to admit it, the emergency room may actually be the right place for her, the only place where she can get an immediate scan of her brain to look for infection or tumor.

On the other hand, she does look awfully well, while people with brain infections usually look awfully sick. And the iffy urine situation sounds very much like she was found to have "dirty urine"—or evidence of street drugs in the urine—on a routine urine screen at her methadone program. And was kicked out of her program. And is very angry, angry enough to be taking who knows what kinds of thought-disordering drugs instead of her methadone. On the other hand, she has been HIV-positive for a long time, and the chances of her coming down with a serious infection are relatively high. Even little things should be taken seriously. But on the other hand, to be perfectly practical, no one short of Jesus himself is likely to persuade her down to the emergency room this afternoon.

We lock eyes for a second.

"You're very angry today, Deborah."

"I went to my doctor, Dr. Schwartz, last week and he says I have 500 T cells. HOW COME YOU SAY I'M SO SICK? I'M A BLACK WOMAN, DOCTOR!"

"Do you think you might feel safer in the emergency room, Deborah, where we can make sure that everything's all right with—"

"OH, NO." She rises to a full height of twelve feet, never taking her eyes off my face. "You don't send me down there for a urine test, they don't do black people's urine." She pauses. "You can just give me eardrops. I'll wait outside."

And out she sweeps, out of the examining room area, out of the waiting room, down the main corridor, out of sight. I write out a prescription for earwax remover, but I know she won't be back for it today. The mention of the emergency room is always a potent deterrent to return.

The next day I call Dr. Schwartz, who hasn't seen Deborah in almost a year, and Mary calls Deborah's aunt, just to check in. Mary has called Deborah's aunt after all of Deborah's bad days in the clinic. We realized long ago that it's all we can really do, short of calling the police. At first Mary cringed at intruding on the private tragedy of one of her senior colleagues like this, but both of them have become quite good at these calls over the years. The amenities are always observed, the subtext never revealed. Deborah is just fine this morning, much calmer, never better. No need to worry about her. Her ear's been bothering her a little, is all. But she's so grateful to us for everything we're doing for her. She talks about us all the time.

We never know exactly how to interpret these conversations, but at least we're reassured that nothing has really changed.

> *July 1991*
> *February 1992*
> *August 1992*
> March 1993

As I dodge through the waiting room to my cubicle at the beginning of the clinic session, an emaciated patient slumped in a wheelchair catches my eye and waggles her fingers at me. A friendly gesture, but I don't recognize either the patient or the older woman sitting next to her, and I am briefly thankful that I won't be the one dealing with them today. My appointment slots are all filled up with revisits, and this patient looks complicated, time-consuming, and sick. She must be new to the clinic, probably newly discharged from the hospital with dozens of loose ends to reweave.

But when, a few hours later, I call out for Deborah Sweet, whom I can't locate anywhere in the waiting room, the older woman of the pair gathers up their belongings and slowly wheels the chair across the room toward me.

Oh, Deborah.

At her last appointment six weeks ago she had been complaining of stomach pain and had lost some weight. ("My ulcer's acting up again.") She had a thin coating of thrush in her mouth and a court date scheduled for the following week. ("You have to write me another letter.") I wrote the letter and encouraged her to take her Diflucan for the fungus that might be creeping from her mouth down into her stomach, idly wondering how much longer this unusual concatenation of fungus and the law was going to continue. Diagnosed with AIDS for almost four years now, Deborah was doing awfully well, with no long hospitalizations or major infections to sap her strength. My suspicions still tended toward her selling rather than ingesting most of her medications, and if I was right her well-being was even more statistically unusual: without treatment most AIDS patients die within a year of their diagnosis. But Deborah was always a statistic unto herself.

The patient being pushed toward me in the wheelchair is wrapped in Deborah's sweater and is holding her handbag. That's all I recognize. The face is a stranger's, hollowed and elongated, one side drooping and a thin stream of saliva tracing a path from the left corner of her mouth to a tissue carefully tucked under her chin. The eyes look up at me mildly. The fingers waggle again.

"Oh, Deborah." I can't say anything else.

The woman pushing Deborah reaches out around the chair and gives me a brisk handshake. "Mrs. Malone," she says. "Deb's aunt. I'm so pleased to meet you at last."

They follow me into the examining room. It's always a tight squeeze in there with a wheelchair, but Mrs. Malone manages neatly, parallel-parking the chair in the corner, adjusting the tissue under Deborah's chin, and settling herself into the chair by the desk.

"What happened?" It isn't the right thing to say, I know, but I can't seem to figure out what is.

"Well, now, Doctor, Deb has had a small stroke." Mrs. Malone leans forward and, like the well-trained nurse she is, gives me a full report. "She's doing OK now, though, and that's a fact. Her appetite is good, and she passes her urine and stool right in the commode if I help her with the transfer. We get her out of bed to chair once or twice a day, her husband and her uncle and I, after her breakfast and after her supper. But Doctor, she's not sleeping at night. That's the real problem. She's not sleeping. Are you, Deb?"

Deborah's eyes widen and she shakes her head a little. With an effort she forces a few sounds out of her mouth that, strangled though they are, I can interpret with no problem: "Don't forget to write me for my Ativan today."

"She does need some medication for sleep, Doctor, and that's a fact. Sit up a little, Deb, you're going to roll right over."

Mrs. Malone gets up to readjust Deborah in the wheelchair, lifting her professionally under the armpits and settling her back against the pillows.

"But, Mrs. Malone, when did this happen? Why didn't you call us? Why didn't you bring her to the hospital?"

"Oh, well now, I'd say it was about a month ago. Yes, that's about it, it was right after her birthday that I noticed her face was drooping a little, and then a few days later she started having trouble with that arm, and then the leg came the next week. But I got her a hospital bed right away, and it has certainly come in handy."

"But, Mrs. Malone . . ."

What do I say? But, Mrs. Malone, what have you done? But, Mrs. Malone, the stepwise progression of a stroke that you describe is a medical emergency? But, Mrs. Malone, she should have had a scan, a neurologist, some blood tests, right away? But, Mrs. Malone, we would have treated her, we would have given her antibiotics right away, in case she has the toxo infection that gives AIDS patients strokes, or possibly syphilis or tuberculosis of the brain; we could have saved her for another month, or six, or twelve, for another court date, another scene in the clinic, another dirty urine at another methadone program. But, Mrs. Malone?

Mrs. Malone is gazing at me calmly, right in the eye, the same gaze that every older nurse has ever gazed at every young flummoxed doctor. Deborah, now slumped over in the chair, eyes closed, is snoring softly through an open mouth.

"I can take good care of my baby now, Doctor. She's had a long fight. She's tired."

"But, Mrs. Malone . . ."

"She can take a CT of the brain next week if you want. Not until next week, though; it's such a struggle getting her down the porch stairs. And there's sixteen more stairs up to her apartment, too. I'm keeping her on the AZT five times daily, is that right? You'll have to sign equipment forms for the hospital bed and commode. Are there any other medications you think she should be taking?"

I make Deborah's CT scan appointment. I write prescriptions for the antibiotics that might have worked a month ago. I write her Ativan prescription. Waking Deborah up, I draw blood from a fat antecubital vein that pops from her skeletal forearm while she watches idly.

"Look, Deborah. A vein in your arm! Remember how hard it used to be to draw your blood?"

She nods slightly, and looks away.

Michael Soto

MARCH 1989

Mary is lurking in the doorway of my examining room, hovering at the edge of my peripheral vision and casting a shadow over the desk.

"*What is it?*" If she would only go away, I could concentrate on the stack of Byzantine disability forms I have come early to the clinic specifically to deal with, but she doesn't move.

"Michael Soto is here," she says for the second time, extending a chart a little farther in my direction.

"I don't know Michael Soto," I say, also for the second time, hastily scribbling a signature on the bottom of a form. "I know Mayra Soto and Sylvia Soto. Those are my Sotos. All I know about Michael is that Medical Records keeps filing his blood slips in Sylvia's chart. That's it. Ask someone else."

The chart lands on my desk with a thud. "Nobody knows Michael Soto. And you're the only one here yet. He's followed in the medical clinic. They made him an appointment to come here this afternoon but they wrote the wrong time on the card again. He's been here since 8 A.M. He's a very nice man. I'm not keeping him waiting any longer."

Our irregular clinic hours confuse everybody. We are an afternoon clinic twice a week and a morning clinic once a week. Patients are told to arrive at 8:30 A.M. on Mondays, or at 1 P.M. on Wednesdays and Thursdays. Doctors switch back and forth from morning to afternoon sessions depending on the rest of their schedule during a given month. The clerks in charge of giving out appointments at the front desk have a hard time keeping it all straight. Most of our patients learn the schedule and automatically correct their appointment cards when a mistake is made. But the new patients referred from other clinics, trusting souls, are occasionally misscheduled into arriving four hours early for an afternoon appointment or four hours late for a morning one.

I look at my watch. It is now about a quarter to one. I have been sincerely looking forward to fetching myself a cup of coffee between the end of my paperwork and the beginning of the afternoon clinic. On the other hand, this Soto has definitely broken all records as far as heroic waits go. His chart is slender. And Mary is annoyed. All good reasons to see him without a murmur of protest, even though it isn't my turn to take a new patient, and he will be my third Soto, which is going to make for a lot of confusion.

"Send him in," I say, feeling virtuous.

"Yes, Doctor." She is definitely annoyed.

Thirty seconds later a pink young man hesitates at my door, grinning diffidently. At first glance he glows with health; on closer inspection, his high color is a little too coarse and brilliant, less like a rose than a salmon hydrangea, or a garish teenage shade of blush, "Foxy Flame" perhaps. The thick purple circles under his eyes clash with his cheeks. When he sits down and lets the smile fade from his face he looks worried, exhausted, and uncomfortable.

"Mr. Soto? Dr. Zuger. How are you doing?"

He grins and nods. "Pretty good."

He doesn't look pretty good. He looks terrible. "Really?"

His grin becomes rueful. "No. Not so good. Actually, pretty terrible. I don't usually look like this. This color, I mean. My wife, she says I look like I'm using her makeup. And the itch, it's terrible. I can't take it anymore. I don't sleep. I haven't slept in seven nights. I went to the clinic downstairs, and they told me to call for an appointment in May. May!" He grins again and shrugs. The haphazard triage habits of the overbooked medical clinic downstairs elicit many reactions; few are as mild and philosophical as this one. I find myself grinning back.

It turns out that Mr. Soto's chart is so appealingly slender because most of it is still in Medical Records. I have only volume III of three volumes, but he proves remarkably adept at re-creating volumes I and II for me. He is thirty-two, a drug user until a few years ago, when he discovered he was HIV-positive and joined a methadone program. He was admitted to the hospital in 1987 with a "regular pneumonia." In 1988 he came down with the most common AIDS-related pneumonia, PCP. His PCP diagnosis was confirmed with a biopsy of his lung. At first he was treated with Bactrim, the usual sulfa-containing antibiotic for PCP: "I told them I was allergic to sulfa, but they said they wanted to see for themselves." People have sued the hospital for less, but Mr. Soto apparently only volunteered a polite "I told you so" after a few very itchy days, and was changed to the alternate drug pentamidine.

Since his discharge from the hospital last December he has been seen a couple of times in the medical clinic by an assortment of hospital interns and residents. One resident gave him prescriptions for AZT and pentamidine to breathe in through a nebulizer at home to prevent the PCP from recurring. Another gave him an antibiotic for bronchitis. A month ago he got an emergency call to come back to the clinic, where a third resident wearing a face mask, whose name Mr. Soto didn't catch, possibly because it wasn't offered, told Mr. Soto that he had come down with tuberculosis. He was given a handful of prescription slips and an X-ray form and told to return in three months. And now here he is, glowing, itchy, and sleepless.

In his chart a scrawled note I can't read very well records this last encounter. Apparently, a sputum specimen sent to the lab a few months earlier, during Mr. Soto's episode of bronchitis, has grown a mycobacterium in culture. Per hospital protocol, the medical clinic was notified immediately. The bacteria that cause TB are mycobacteria, but so are ten or fifteen other more benign microorganisms, many of which don't cause human disease and don't have to be treated. It usually takes weeks to months of growth in the laboratory before one mycobacterium can be distinguished from another.

The masked man who showered Mr. Soto with tuberculosis pills had the right idea—concern for the public health mandates that a mycobacterium is assumed to be tuberculous until it is proved otherwise. But our hero left the job half done, the second part being the somewhat less swashbuckling responsibility of keeping an eye on both patient and mycobacterium during the first few months of treatment. Mycobacteria that grow up to be distant cousins of tuberculosis need no treatment, while tuberculosis usually requires months to years of an

assortment of drugs. And patients with AIDS are notorious for developing reactions to even the most benign
medications. When Mr. Soto takes off his shirt he
becomes living proof of this medical fact.

"Pretty bad, huh?" He is grinning again, while I am
absorbed in a close inspection of his neck, trying to figure
out if he has three separate rashes or only two. On his
face, forearms, and chest the "Foxy Flame" effect proves to
come from a lawn of tiny fluid-filled blisters, while
on his back and trunk sweeping scabbed-over scratch
marks crisscross a background of flat pinkish splotches. I
decide it doesn't really matter how many rashes he has,
the major question of the morning being exactly how
unnecessary they all are.

On the phone, the technician in the microbiology
lab is more than helpful: Mr. Soto's mycobacterium was
identified several weeks ago as an *M. gordonae,* a complete
nonentity of an organism not worth a second thought, let
alone a collection of rashes like this.

"So that means you can stop taking the pills for the
tuberculosis, it was all a false alarm. Just give me a second
to write this all down and I'll go over them with you."

"That means I don't take anymore the INH, the
rifampin, the pyra . . . pyrazinamide and the vitamin?"

I stop writing in his chart and stare at him. Not only
does this Michael Soto come early to appointments, wait
where others would leave, shrug where others would sue,
and recite a coherent medical history, but he also knows
the names and purposes of all his medicines. At the look

on my face he grins again. "My wife says I gotta know what I'm taking."

"Yes, well, that's wonderful. She's right. Everybody should know what they're taking. Look, can you come see me here in this clinic from now on? Can you come in next week so we can make sure everything's getting better and take care of a few other routine things?"

"Next week?" His eyes widen a little, and his smile seems to broaden and suffuse his whole weirdly fluorescent face with light. "Oh, yes. I will be here."

I am under strict orders to send patients like him back down to the medical clinic, where the residents get their experience in taking care of patients with AIDS. ("You know, not the, er, problem patients," the director of the medical clinic said at our meeting. "The simpler ones. The, er, friendly ones. Those are the ones we want for the residents.")

But the residents in the medical clinic don't deserve Mr. Soto. And I do.

March 1989

February 1990

I know it's going to be a Soto day the moment I round the corner and head down the long corridor toward the clinic door. On Soto days the small neat figures of Michael Soto and his wife are always there ahead of me, sitting side by side on a bench in the corridor outside the entrance to the waiting room, always early, always smiling and nodding as I approach. I always stop in the corridor for a second. "How are you?" He always grins and bobs his head. "Pretty good."

It is turning out that almost every week for the last year has had a Soto day, because Mr. Soto is in fact almost never pretty good. Somewhere between his neck and waist he is almost always pretty terrible. He has a set of remarkably complicated lungs that have been tormenting him for years, and his HIV infection has only made things worse. He was an asthmatic child, began to smoke as a teenager, and apparently had the kind of PCP that ravages the lung tissue, destroying its natural balloonlike elasticity and leaving large, flabby, useless pouches behind. Even with a normal immune system these pieces of lung would be at continuous risk of infection; with the flimsy Soto immune defenses, they are rarely free of it.

Sometimes he is coming down with bronchitis, sometimes with pneumonia, sometimes he is relapsing, sometimes recrudescing. Whatever it is, he is always much too polite to complain. He seems to feel it is disloyal to keep getting sick in the face of all my diligence, much less to complain about his symptoms. This uncommon trait is proving to be a surprisingly formidable obstacle to the efficient delivery of medical care.

"So!" I say after his chart finally works its way to the front of my stack and he is sitting in the examining room. "How are you feeling?"

"Good! Pretty good!"

"Really good?"

"Yes, really, much better!"

"You're taking the new antibiotics? Did they give you a rash? Did they give you a stomachache?"

"No, they're fine, no problem at all. I feel good!"

"It looks like you've lost a little weight again."

"I wore my sneakers today, they're lighter than the shoes last week. And last week I had a coat on, too."

"Are you still coughing?"

"Today it's better. Much better."

"How about the fever?"

"This morning, so far, it didn't come back!"

Aha.

"So you had fever yesterday? Last night?"

"No, not really. Not too much. Anyway, today it's much better!"

"So you feel better than last week?"

"Better!"

"Much better?"

"Better!"

At this point I move on to examine his chest, although I've begun to realize that here too I might as well save my energy. While he refuses to complain, his lungs never stop. When I listen to his chest with a stethoscope I never hear the whish-whoosh of healthy airways. His lungs wheeze and trill like an organ even when he really does seem to be feeling well, undercutting his constant cheer with their constant whining, particularly that high annoying squeak near his right shoulder blade that never goes away. His chest X rays are uniformly disastrous, so distorted by the scars of his past infections that they imply he is on his deathbed. He never is.

"I'm fine. Really. Fine."

"Your X ray looks terrible."

"But I feel better!"

"Much better?"

"Better!"

In medical school students are taught to record the patient's complaints (the "subjective" portion of the medical assessment) and then to confirm them with the physical exam and laboratory findings (the "objective" portion). No course mentions what to do when the two portions completely cancel each other out. In the absence of formal policy I have proceeded by instinct and random hazard. Sometimes I believe Mr. Soto's lungs and give him new antibiotics, more antibiotics, better antibiotics. Sometimes I believe Mr. Soto and send him home without. Sometimes I try to enlist his wife's collaboration, but she has declined all invitations into the examining room with a smile, a shake of the head, and the apologetic sweep of hand to mouth of the non-English-speaker.

Last week I had an inspiration and let Mr. Soto sit in the examining room while I did a little paperwork. After fifteen minutes he began to cough, to our great mutual relief. He was spared the disrespectful necessity of telling me straight out that my carefully chosen antibiotics of the last visit had done him no good at all, and I was given a little actual information on the state of his health.

"Still coughing, I see."

He coughed some more.

"Doesn't seem like that antibiotic really did the trick, eh?"

Cough.

I wrote him a prescription for the one antibiotic I could think of that he hadn't taken in a while and isn't allergic to, and sent him home.

This week my heart sinks as I glimpse the Sotos on their bench far down the corridor. He doesn't have an appointment scheduled for today, so he must be feeling worse. And I've run out of antibiotics. As I draw near they both nod from their perch on the bench in the corridor as always. In the dim light he looks marvelous, the picture of health, but while he bobs a cheerful greeting, his pretty, plump, black-haired wife looks at me unsmiling and shakes her head a little. Sure enough, in the examining room he is, once again, Foxy Flame.

"You are now allergic to every major oral antibiotic known to man."

He grins. "I know. It's terrible."

"When did you stop taking them?"

"Three days ago."

"How are you feeling?"

"Better!"

"How is the fever?"

"I think there was a little fever," he says delicately, disowning it. He is, in fact, almost 103°. When I listen to his chest, alarming atonal noises come out of his left lung. His right lung is squeaking like a cicada. I can hear it even without the stethoscope. (And I can hear what it's saying, too: "Don't belieeeeve him, help meeeeee, pleeeease.") I am willing to stretch almost every rule in the book for this saintly, pleasant, red man, but I have run out of tricks. I know he hates the hospital, all our patients do. But this latest allergy has me checkmated. There's nothing else I can do but admit him to the hospital to receive an intravenous antibiotic that he isn't allergic to.

I explain, and for the first time that I can remember, he stops smiling.

"It's terrible there," he says so bitterly I barely recognize him. "I don't go back in there. I do everything you say, everything. But not back there."

"Look, just for a few days." I tend to say this even when I don't mean it, but in his case I really think it's true. What he has isn't one of the untreatable life-threatening infections AIDS patients get. It's just a simple ordinary pneumonia that I can't treat with pills. If he had private insurance I could call a visiting nurse service to give him antibiotic infusions at home, but none of these services will accept Medicaid payments.

He looks away from me, grim and glowing, lips compressed. I hadn't known him during his hospitalization. Was it a dying roommate, a callous intern, a fortnight of interrupted sleep, or the glut of tests that did it?

"They scare my wife. They tell her I'm dying. They say I got six months. She break down, you know, break down, breakdown. They scare everybody there. Look, it's two years. I'm not dying. I don't go back to hear that again."

Well-meaning people in the hospital are always trying to get newly diagnosed AIDS patients to face facts. What they said and what he has remembered may be two different things, but I imagine he got the tenor of the interaction quite accurately.

"Why don't you go outside and bring her in. I'll try to explain to her myself. OK?"

But when he comes back into the examining room five minutes later he is alone, as always, and grinning and shrugging, as always. "She says I gotta do what you say. She says she knew already I had to go in. She says she'll be OK. She says I'll be OK."

"Sounds like she knows everything."

"She knows."

When the messenger comes to take him down to the emergency room for admission I find myself walking alongside the wheelchair like an anxious parent, full of last-minute advice. "Don't forget to tell them about your allergies!" He nods patiently and waves.

March 1989
February 1990

October 1990

"He says what?"

"He says he feels terrible."

"You're sure? I don't believe you. This is Mr. Soto saying that?"

"That's what I *said*. I told you already. Terrible. Like he's going to die, he says. Now, what should I do? Does he get like this often?"

The nurse on the phone has known Mr. Soto for only a couple of weeks and doesn't understand why I am having such a hard time understanding English. I am in her office barely three minutes later, watching him shake like a leaf.

"T-t-terrible!" He can barely get the words out. His fair skin, which I have previously seen run through the entire red end of the spectrum, is now a pale, translucent green. His hair is soaked. Kate, the nurse who called me, has haphazardly piled a few blankets on top of him. "He came in like this," she says. "This is his week two visit: Symptom-Oriented Physical Exam and Blood Tests. He says it started last week. How in the world am I supposed to code these chills?"

Kate is the nurse in charge of enrolling patients in the hospital's AIDS-related research protocols. The hospital where I work, like thirty or forty others across the country, is part of a federal research network called the Aids Clinical Trials Group (ACTG), the purpose of which is to carry out large-scale studies of new AIDS drugs. This network of hospitals all collaborating in the same drug research has been organized with the best of intentions: the more patients that are enrolled into studies of new AIDS drugs, the more quickly the safety and effectiveness of these agents can be assessed. However, large-scale collaboration makes for a lot of small-scale annoyances, all of which Kate can discuss at some length. She reserves a special hatred for the form on which she has to assign a numerical code to each symptom a patient develops on medication so that all the information can be entered into a centralized computer.

I sent Mr. Soto to talk to Kate about a research protocol about a month ago. He has been on AZT for almost two years. AZT is still the only anti-HIV drug on the market, but a few alternatives are in the works. All the experts now suspect that with AIDS, as with any chronic infection, alternating a few effective drugs or combining them will turn out to be the best way to suppress the infection. And ACTG Protocol 117 is Mr. Soto's only chance at this point to get a shot at DDI, a cousin of AZT's that seems to be a promising treatment alternative.

People who enroll in Protocol 117 are given a packet of pills and a box of little paper envelopes filled with powder to take home. They take the pills and drink the powder dissolved in water. Half of them will be taking AZT and drinking bicarbonate of soda; the other half will be drinking DDI and taking sugar pills. In the way of research, so as not to prejudice the results of the study, only a computer knows who is taking what. Pills and envelopes are ingested and refilled, ingested and refilled, blood is tested, symptoms are coded. At regular intervals, the central computer looks deep inside itself and analyzes the study data pouring into its disks from all over the country. If one medication has made patients do better or live longer than the other, the study is stopped, the results are announced, and one more tiny piece of the mosaic of AIDS is set in grout.

Mr. Soto listened to my explanation of Protocol 117 with his customary polite interest. He had been feeling well and his routine visits had been down to once a month for quite a while. I felt a certain inclination not to rock the boat by changing his medications around, but one of the two Sotos is clearly a natural gambler. When he came back into the examining room after the usual outside conference, it was with the usual nod, smile, and shrug. Forty-five minutes later he was in Kate's office, looking over a copy of the ten-page consent form he has to sign.

And now, two weeks later, something is terribly wrong.

We get him down to the emergency room in record time, Kate pushing and me pulling a stretcher with a broken left front wheel that makes it keep careening into the corridor walls. Every time we bump into a wall Mr. Soto groans, and Mrs. Soto following behind carrying his jacket groans, and Kate and I wince and groan too. In the ER he is unceremoniously taken out of our hands. The triage nurse onto whose overflowing clipboard Mr. Soto lands allows me about thirty seconds of attention, barely enough time to cover his allergies, let alone his lungs. I don't even bother bringing up the medical and legal complexities of a near fatal reaction to an unlicensed, experimental drug. Kate, poor thing, is going to have to deal with the Adverse Event form, enough to make a person cry.

Mrs. Soto stands by the stretcher, ferociously holding Mr. Soto's hand. The chief ER doctor I corner with my theories of sepsis, adrenal failure, and recurrent pneumonia is calm and not very interested. He tells me not to worry, that all the bases will be covered. I recognize a phrase specifically designed to urge me off the premises. I am not only unnecessary in the ER, I am *de trop*, occupying valuable square footage on which another stretcher could be placed. I retreat to my office, where I spend the rest of the day deeply wishing I hadn't rocked Mr. Soto's boat.

It is all I can do to force myself back down to the ER before I go home that night. I have heard nothing all day. He could be dead—they seldom call from the ER when this happens, and if Mrs. Soto won't risk her English in person, she's unlikely to do so on the phone. He could have been transferred by now to intensive care, where he is bound to undergo all sorts of gruesome and painful tests (all my fault, all my fault), he could be on a respirator (his lungs could never survive that), on dialysis, in surgery for an acute abdominal catastrophe from that cursed DDI. I call Kate, but she's not at her desk. I contemplate going home without seeing him.

I find myself in the ER. Mr. Soto is on a stretcher sandwiched between others way toward the back of the room. To his right an emaciated elderly lady is screaming for the police. To his left a patient whose face I recognize from our clinic is dozing, a face mask dangling from one ear. The noise is intense. Mrs. Soto and Kate are squeezed in alongside Mr. Soto's stretcher, watching him eat a giant helping of arroz con pollo out of a Tupperware container.

"Better!" He doesn't even wait for the question. "Much better!"

I look at Kate. She shrugs. "They gave him some methadone," she says. "His wife told someone he was withdrawing."

I look at him. He nods, mouth full, swallows. "It was terrible," he says. "It was the same thing that happened when they made me take the rifampin, and the program, they had to give me more methadone. She figure it out, and she tell the nurse, and now, I'm much better!" Another big grin.

Withdrawing! Of course. He has been withdrawing from methadone. Some drugs, like rifampin, stimulate the liver enzymes that break down methadone; others prevent the stomach from absorbing methadone. Either can make addicts who have been stable and comfortable on a methadone dose for years suddenly start to withdraw. DDI is too new a drug to have had all of its interactions fully evaluated. But, if any of us had been thinking logically, we would have remembered that the powder component of Protocol 117 is a strong antacid. Whether it contains DDI or not, it can wreak havoc on the absorptive powers of the stomach. It has probably been preventing Mr. Soto from absorbing his methadone. You'd think someone might have warned us—but that, of course, is what research is for, to make the warnings.

Kate is shaking her head. "Now what?" Visions of Symptom/Complaint forms, Adverse Event forms, Withdrawal from Study forms are clearly furrowing her brow. She has been working with research patients for a long time and knows how jittery and unforgiving a person is apt to become when he signs a ten-page consent form, ingests a quantity of unlabeled substances, and then spends an afternoon at death's door. She can't imagine that Mr. Soto, having weathered one Adverse Event, is likely to stay in the study for more. I, with more Soto experience under my belt, am not so sure.

"We can always fix it so the methadone and the powder don't reach his stomach at the same time. And get him a little more methadone. That should take care of it. Or he can always quit being in the study, if he wants, and go back to the AZT."

Lightheaded with relief though I am, I am trying to sound completely impartial. Staying in the study, where there is a 50 percent chance that he is getting DDI, will almost certainly be better for him in the long run. But he has to make the decision for himself, not to please me. I can't read his face, and his mouth is too full for him to talk. Mrs. Soto begins to shake her head and talk soft Spanish emphatically into his ear. He chews, swallows, chews, swallows.

"She says I gotta stay in," he finally announces when he can talk, snapping the lid back on the Tupperware. "I maybe think so too."

March 1989
February 1990
October 1990

May 1992

"Pretty good!" Dressed for the spring in Bermuda shorts and loafers, Mr. Soto lets his bare legs swing cheerfully against the examining table. It is the last saint's day of the parochial school year, and his daughter, Melissa, is outside in the corridor with her mother, stroking a dilapidated Barbie doll and displaying the familial talent for patient waiting. When I first met his only child she was a rotund three-year-old. Now she is six, skinny, and despite her vacation day, decked out in school plaid. In the examining room her father is clearly poised for a rapid departure from the clinic out into the spring. I glance down to his chart for today's temperature and have a hard time believing it.

"A mistake." He nods confidently. "That machine is terrible, always broken." In fact, the electronic thermometer used by the nurses has always seemed to be remarkably sturdy and accurate. I dig up a stray paper thermometer in a desk drawer and put it in his mouth. He is, in fact, 103.6°, exactly as advertised.

He shrugs, but his smile dims. "Maybe another mistake? I feel good."

He does look pretty well. He has lost two or three pounds in the year he has been taking his

Protocol 117 medicines, but he is still ten pounds heavier than before he started them. His skin is clear, and his lungs are in their springtime hiatus of clarity between the bronchitis of the winter and the humidity-induced asthma of the summer. I listen to them again. Some echoes of the usual complaints, fewer than usual. His abdomen—fine. His heart—fine. His arms, legs, fingers, toes—all fine. No headache. No blurry vision. The back of his eyes where infection sometimes lurks—fine. His mouth and teeth—fine. After fifteen minutes of diligent inspection, all I can find is a walnut-sized lump in his neck behind his left collarbone that I don't remember feeling before.

"How long has this been here?"

"Maybe a week."

"Does it hurt?"

"Maybe a little, when he swells up."

"When it swells up?"

"Sometimes it seems like he's getting bigger and bigger every day."

"Are the others getting bigger too?" He has small lymph nodes all over his neck, but these are so common in patients with AIDS that unless one node is distinguished from its fellows by size, tenderness, or asymmetry, we usually pay them little attention.

"No, just him."

"You know, I had a patient who used to give his lymph nodes names. You know, Harry, Miguel . . ." Why am I saying this? Mr. Soto nods, but clearly he doesn't think it's very funny, and neither, suddenly, do I.

I send him off for a chest X ray. This time, unlike all the other times he has headed down to Radiology with a fever and an X-ray requisition, he goes with my devout hopes that something will be wrong with his lungs on the films he brings back up. A nice simple pneumonia located in some region of his chest I can't hear well with the stethoscope would be my abnormality of choice. One of Mr. Soto's pneumonias is a treatable, self-limited infection, a normal infection. Things that infiltrate lymph nodes, making them swell and hurt, are not. These are the much-feared opportunistic infections and tumors of AIDS, caused by weird, misshapen, microbial and cellular misfits. These creatures cannot survive in the presence of normal immune systems, but they show up in immunocompromised systems with moving vans and suitcases and never leave. Antibiotics and chemotherapy will drive them out as far as the back lawn, but no farther. They always linger, ready to reappear if treatment isn't continued. Mr. Soto has been very lucky so far to have escaped with only one of them, his episode of PCP three and a half years ago.

I'm not really surprised when there is no sign of pneumonia on the X ray he brings back upstairs. Instead, it shows an unmistakable chain of swollen lymph nodes snaking all the way down the center of his chest. That small one in the neck is no aberration. It is an early outpost of invasion, sentinel to an army of invaders with suitcases in hand.

The lymph node in his neck has to be biopsied. Looking at a fragment of it under the microscope is the only efficient way of figuring out what kind of invaders are marching in, and what kind of treatment is most likely to keep them at bay for a while. Unfortunately, as easy as the node is to see, feel, anesthetize, and aim a needle at, it couldn't be located in a worse place for arranging a biopsy.

The neck is a jointly owned surgical territory, its lumps fair game for many surgical services—but all the surgeons in the clinics we deal with have an infuriating tendency to remember their manners when our patients show up in their waiting rooms. Mr. Soto's loafers thump against the examining table as I stare at his chart and mentally tick off the alternatives. When we send patients to the general surgery clinic for a lymph-node biopsy, the residents usually send them on to the ear, nose, and throat clinic. When we refer directly to the ENT clinic, the residents there tend to bounce people off for a consultation with Surgical Oncology, who usually like to refer on to Cytology. Of course, there was also the time a creative ENT resident actually sent a patient over to the cardiothoracic clinic for a biopsy of the nodes within his chest instead of the ones on his neck. This considerably more dangerous and uncomfortable procedure unquestionably belonged in another guy's turf.

As stones are sent skipping across the bay, so our patients skim the surface of the surgical clinics. It's not that these resident surgeons—the only ones available to our patients with Medicaid—outright refuse to operate on AIDS patients. It's just that no one seems to be counseling them to fight their instincts to duck. It wouldn't be so frustrating were it not for the fact that each appointment takes weeks, sometimes months, to schedule. By the time a biopsy is actually arranged, the patients have often become so sick from whatever it is in that lymph node that they have been put in the hospital, where they become some other surgeon's problem. My last patient with a lump in her neck languished for a couple of months between appointments until someone—could it have been a surgeon in the breast clinic?—finally caved in and did the biopsy. Perhaps I should actually send Mr. Soto directly to the breast clinic? That would be a first. If he only had some other kind of insurance I could send him to a private surgeon and have the biopsy done in a flash. But private surgeons don't accept Medicaid payments that barely cover their afternoon coffee, let alone their overhead. If I took some kind of course or other I could probably do the biopsy myself. A snip, a stitch—how hard could it be? I'll have to look into it.

Mary makes some phone calls to the head nurses of the various surgical clinics. Everyone has a five-week wait for an appointment. We decide to gamble on the breast clinic. ("Better tell them straight out it isn't a breast," says the head nurse there. "You never know.") I get a consultation form out of the drawer and begin to fill it out. Mr. Soto's loafers bang against the examining table. The afternoon is getting on.

"I'm sorry this all took so long."

"OK, no problem."

"What were you going to do today?"

"Melissa and me, we're gonna fish."

"Fish?"

"On City Island. In the summer we get blues. Not so many fish now, but she makes me take her."

He embarks on an enthusiastic discussion of pier fishing off the coast of the Bronx. Usually I love to hear him talk in paragraphs instead of phrases, but suddenly I am barely listening. I have filled out a consultation form with a short paragraph summarizing Mr. Soto's medical history and the reason I am sending him to the breast clinic ("biopsy of supraclavicular mass IN THE NECK"). When I begin to copy his name and number from his clinic card onto the top of form, I find myself staring at the billing code on the top of his card. All Medicaid patients have "031" embossed in that slot. But here he has an "023" by his name.

"Has something happened to your Medicaid?"

"No. No problem with the Medicaid."

"You've got a funny number here."

"That's my new card. I just got it. I got Medicare now too."

It completely slipped my mind that he has passed his two years with a chronic disabling illness, thus qualifying for Medicare. He is an insured person. He is welcome in private surgical offices. He has lived long enough to graduate from the Medicaid clinics. We don't mark this event very frequently with our patients, who seldom survive long enough after an AIDS diagnosis to achieve Medicare coverage. I rip up the consult form and throw the shreds over him like confetti. Fifteen minutes later he has an appointment with a private oncological surgeon for the next day and is heading out down the hall. Melissa has promised to bring me a fish.

March 1989
February 1990
October 1990
May 1992

August 1992

Waves of heat shimmer against the side of the building. Inside the clinic, patients wilt in the sunny waiting room while the windowless examining rooms are dank and icy. Mr. Soto, shirtless and trouserless, is shivering on my examining table while I am, as usual, peering at a portion of his back with my penlight, trying to figure out his new hue.

My heart sank when he walked in. Two weeks ago he was a normal color. Today his face and forearms are a glowing neon salmon.

"I don't believe it. It must be one of those new antibiotics. But we haven't changed anything for weeks now."

"Months. Since June."

"Months. Usually you react right away. And this rash is funny, so faint on your stomach, so bad on your arms and neck, not like usual."

"I feel good. This time it doesn't itch."

No, he has none of the usual scratch marks on his back today. In fact, he has no marks at all. I step back for a broader perspective. This is more of a wash effect than a rash, really, more of a glow, a blush, a burn. A burn.

"Ha."

He looks at me.

"Sunburn. This is a sunburn. You went fishing and you have a sunburn." I put my penlight back in my pocket with dignity.

Broad smile. "Yeah, I did a little fishing. I forgot to say. I got you fooled. This time, it's the fishing medicine!" Big laugh. Mr. Soto loves his own jokes.

The state of his health has had us both on a roller-coaster ride since the afternoon I arranged his appointment with the surgeon for his lymph-node biopsy. In the ten days between the scheduling and the performing of the biopsy he went downhill with dizzying speed. He lost almost fifteen pounds and his nightly fevers climbed to 105° with drenching sweats. His red blood cell count went down ten points, so low that the surgeon suggested he get a blood transfusion before the procedure.

The biopsy itself went without incident. Three days later, pale and sweaty, Mr. Soto came to clinic to find out the results. I wasn't entirely surprised when Mrs. Soto left her bench in the hallway that afternoon and crept into the examining room behind him. Her instincts were always infallible. I could feel her huge black eyes boring into the back of my head as I called the pathology lab.

I knew that all the preliminary tests on the lymph node had been negative. The results of more important tests, which require several extra days for the tissue to be fixed and stained, would be ready that afternoon. If he had a lymphoma, my great fear, it would show up only on these later tests. This cancer of the lymph nodes that becomes increasingly common in longer-term survivors of AIDS was the least treatable of all the major possibilities for his illness. I was trying to be realistic. Mr. Soto had already had more than his statistical share of treatable infections.

The pathologist was pleasant and definite on the phone. She had just finished reading his slides and remembered them well. "Granuloma and AFB," she said. "That's it."

"You're sure? No lymphoma?"

"Granuloma. AFB. Loads of AFB. That's it."

Granuloma are the clusters of infection-fighting cells that form in a person with tuberculosis. AFB (acid-fast bacilli) are the TB organisms themselves.

"You're sure?"

"I'm sure, I'm sure. You think they pay me to make mistakes?"

I took a deep breath. Mr. Soto had just been handed another reprieve. He had a diagnosis of tuberculosis of the lymph nodes. A treatable infection, the best outcome that could have been imagined. For about six weeks we wouldn't know the final diagnosis—the bacteria the pathologist saw under the microscope could be the ones usually associated with human tuberculosis, or they could be MAI—*M. avium intracellulare*—an organism that causes a lot of tuberculosis in patients with AIDS and very little in people with normal immune systems. Regular tuberculosis could be treated pretty easily; MAI was harder to treat, but a few months earlier a powerful new antibiotic with good results against it had been released. Mr. Soto had timed his illness superbly. Either way, he now had a fighting chance that this crisis too would pass.

When I turned around, Mrs. Soto was beaming and clutching his hand before I had a chance to say a word.

He got worse before he got better. Not wanting to take any chances, I started him on a regimen of medications that would treat both kinds of tuberculosis. It was shaped and reshaped by his allergies. Eventually I had to start giving him antibiotic shots three times a week because I ran out of pill alternatives. His medication list was full of drugs that were notorious for causing upset stomachs and general misery among TB patients in the early 1960s and had largely been replaced by newer, better tolerated ones. But bizarrely, Mr. Soto began to thrive on these old standbys. His fevers and chills slowly disappeared. That sentinel lymph node near his collarbone shrank, as did the nodes on his chest X ray. He regained a little weight, although he remained about forty pounds lighter than when we first met.

The good news I have for him today is that the bacteria in his lymph node have finally been identified as MAI. Most of those drugs I dug out of the old textbooks for him are no longer necessary. All he needs is the newest drug, clarithromycin, and one or two others. The rest I can keep in reserve in case of allergy—I always try to cover myself like this when he's concerned.

His smile broadens as I go down the list with him, lightening his daily load.

"No more PAS, OK?"

"OK!"

"No more cycloserine, OK?"

"OK!"

"No more shots, OK?"

"Ya!"

"So that leaves . . . ?"

"So that leaves Biaxin, two; Myambutol, three; Lamprene, one—all together in the morning."

"Exactly right." As a parent with a mathematically inclined four-year-old, so am I with this prodigy of pill-taking. I love to watch him calculate, and he never lets me down. He can add medications and subtract them, he can double his doses or put them on hold, he can remember what he took when and remind me of what I told him to stop for a few days and then forgot to write down. There is no chance that he will go home this afternoon encased in that small cloud of confusion I often see forming over other patients' heads, ingest the pills that he should stop and stop the ones that are keeping him alive. With Mr. Soto my every whim is fulfilled to the letter.

When his wife appears at my door a few minutes after he says good-bye, I imagine she is just making sure of the medicine changes. I have long suspected her to be at least as pharmaceutically gifted as he is, if not more so. She beams and hands over a heavy shopping bag. Presumably the pills he doesn't need any more?

"His *medicinas?*"

She shakes her head and vanishes. Inside the shopping bag is a plastic bag, which contains another plastic bag, which contains a wet mass of brown paper.

Shortly thereafter, a place for my bluefish is grudgingly made in the refrigerator the nurses use for their lunches. No one in that clinic, least of all those nurses, will ever learn how much I hate fish.

March 1989
February 1990
October 1990
May 1992
August 1992

December 1992

"So, what's new? Doing any ice fishing?"

No answer.

"Hm?"

"Oh. I don't know."

"No fishing?"

Mr. Soto shrugs, shakes his head, swings his legs against the examining table, and refuses to meet my eye.

"Are you feeling all right?"

Another shrug, a tiny nod.

"Pretty good? Terrible? What's up?"

No answer. A shrug, a shadow of a grin.

Something is wrong here, and I suddenly know what it is.

"Did you see the lawyer?"

Small nod.

"And get all the papers?"

Small nod.

I knew it would be this bad, but it had to be done. The Sotos have been coming to the clinic for almost four years now. Other patients and their families besiege us with plans and demands, but those two ask for nothing. The others need cases of Ensure, need ambulette service, need hospital beds; they need their benefits, their Medicaid, their medication; they need the lawyer, the social worker, the dietitian, right away, today; they need need need. But the Sotos sit quietly side by side on their bench in the corridor, out of the waiting room, away from the rest. They even politely refuse the free carfare the clinic provides—they walk to the hospital from their apartment on the Grand Concourse and then walk home again.

About once a year I have pressed an appointment with our clinic social worker on Mr. Soto. He has always refused. He saw the dietitian once, accepted four cans of Ensure, and never asked for more. He seems to shudder at any mention of the lawyer who helps our patients make custody arrangements for minor children. When I tentatively take over the role of social worker, nurse, or lawyer myself, the answer is always the same: "It's OK. We'll take care of it ourselves. It's OK. Anyway, I feel good!"

At our weekly clinic staff meetings, a chilly silence now greets my reports on Mr. Soto. Nobody else knows him very well. He has not made confidants of the nurses who like to monitor the patients' emotional and coping responses to their illness, or the social workers who specialize in counseling dying patients and their families. My periodic attempts to shoo him into the counseled mainstream are recognized for the feeble gestures they are. "He's in denial," someone will pointedly say every once in a while. "Somebody should do something."

I guess somebody should. I guess we're both in denial, and maybe it's the place to be. I can't help feeling that something quite out of my control has been keeping Mr. Soto alive for this long—he has now survived longer after an AIDS diagnosis than almost any other patient followed in the clinic. A little denial can apparently be a very potent tonic.

Still, I have to admit that by some standards his case has become an embarrassment. When I took a moment to leaf through his chart last month, I winced. Nowhere to be found were any of the usual well-intentioned documents designed to smooth a patient's progress into the next world—no documentation of his desired resuscitation status, for instance; no living will setting out what he will and will not accept in the way of intensive care; no health-care proxy form. No clear-cut plan for Melissa's future. No prearranged funeral director. No social work notes. No mention of his wife's HIV status. ("She's fine. We take care of it. She's OK.") Some stupid notes about fish.

I had forgotten until I paged through his chart that when I first met him in 1989 he had weighed 181 pounds. With every major disaster he has shed weight that is never fully regained. At his last visit he weighed 126 pounds (with shoes, no coat). And meanwhile, here are my notes chirping blithely on. "Doing well on MAI meds . . . "Doing well, bronchitis resolved . . ." "Feeling very well, nausea much improved . . ." He might have nothing more than a few random infections diagnosed and treated, he might have all the time in the world. Many trees in this chart, but no forest; many fish, no ocean. I have been successfully ignoring the bigger picture for years.

When I closed his chart I realized it was time to end this little *folie à deux*. If I could no longer find the words to help him number his days, someone else would have to take over. At the end of his last visit, I delivered both Sotos over to our bilingual social worker Paul without asking permission. I shut the door on the three of them and waited for the fallout.

And here it is. He is drooping on the examining table, staring at the floor. His lungs have begun to misbehave again, and I can hear a little rhythmic wheeze with each exhaled breath. His loafers bang against the examining table.

"How did it go?"

An eyebrow shoots up and he shrugs a little at the floor. His hair is tousled, his jeans and turtleneck clean and ironed. I suddenly notice that his clothes fit him perfectly. No wonder that massive weight loss has bypassed my conscious mind. His complexion is clear and ruddy.

One of his MAI medications is a phenazine dye that tends to turn people a strange pinkish-gray, but Mr. Soto, ever idiosyncratic, has been dyed into rosy health. "It was OK. I got all the papers at home. But it upset her a lot."

"Your wife."

"She got real upset. She don't like to talk about it."

"It's hard to talk about."

"She wants me to take all the machines, you know, the breathing machine, the heart-pump machine . . ."

"And what do you think about all the machines?"

"I don't know. I think that maybe I want to take the machines too. But he, the social worker guy, he says no, think some more."

Patients with terminal diseases are not supposed to elect long, hopeless stays attached to machinery in intensive care.

"The guy, he says the machines just make things worse. He says, when you get very sick, nothing help. But you know, I been so sick, so sick! And look, now I feel good. So the guy, I don't believe him."

He pauses.

"You think I should take the machines?"

This is my cue gently to reinforce everything he has been told about the hopelessness of his disease. I open my mouth, but nothing really comes to mind. He's heard all my usual sentences already. He has enough sense to know what I know, that no preparations really prepare. When the time comes he and his wife will do the right thing. In 1988 he was told he had six months to live. One commuted sentence per lifetime is probably enough.

He is looking up at me now, grinning, shrugging. The eyebrow still cocks at its most rueful angle. "Don't worry. We'll take care of it. Anyway, today I feel good!"

But suddenly he looks ill and tired to me, shrunken and flushed, like someone with a chronic incurable disease.

March 1989
February 1990
October 1990
May 1992
August 1992
December 1992

May 1993

Until this year I never bothered to write a list recapitulating Mr. Soto's diagnoses in his chart every time I saw him ("36-year-old Hispanic male, AIDS diagnosed 11/88, recurrent bronchitis, pneumonia, MAI 5/92 . . ."). Until this year I could carry his case in my head, a story I knew as well as my name. But lately he is accumulating new diagnoses almost weekly. They chase him down one after another, as random and relentless as boulders tumbling down a hill. I can't keep them straight in my mind. I have to write them down.

One day during the winter he showed up with a blinding headache and signs of meningitis. He turned out to have an infected sinus deep within his skull, dangerously close to the brain. He got dramatically better on sinus medication, only to arrive in clinic two weeks later limp as a piece of cooked spaghetti, suddenly a diabetic on the verge of coma. Insulin made him feel much better for a month, then he suddenly lost all energy, his blood pressure ran dangerously low, his serum sodium and potassium went all awry. On replacement adrenal hormones he felt "100 percent better" for all of ten days, when he began to cough again.

I make his diagnoses, but I can't remember them all. Maybe I don't want to. I carry Mr. Soto on a card in my pocket now, and in every note in his chart I carefully redefine him. He has become a children's memory game: aseptic meningitis; aseptic meningitis and sphenoid sinusitis; aseptic meningitis, sphenoid sinusitis, and insulin-dependent diabetes; aseptic meningitis, sphenoid sinusitis, insulin-dependent diabetes, and adrenal insufficiency; aseptic meningitis, sphenoid sinusitis, insulin-dependent diabetes, adrenal insufficiency, and presumed PCP. And relapsed MAI. And relapsed sinusitis.

"So. How are you feeling?"

"Pretty good!"

After so many years, I slice through his layers of politeness with swift and reckless shears.

"I don't believe you. Tell me the truth."

"No, really! Pretty good. The fever went."

"Went completely?"

"I think so. Last night, 99. And no sweating."

"The headache?"

"It went too."

"How's the pain?"

His spleen, swollen and congested from the burden of so many chronic infections, has been throbbing in the left side of his abdomen for some years now.

"The same. Terrible."

"Does the Percocet still help or do you need something stronger?"

"No, the Percocet is OK. But I need some more."

"OK. How about all the others?"

Like any longtime couple, we have evolved a language of our own—a remarkably primitive one, it turns out. We use five or ten concrete nouns (fever and headache, cough and sweat), no abstractions, two adjectives (good and terrible), one adverb (pretty), and about seventy-five brand names. Between the medications he takes and the ones to which he is allergic, Mr. Soto has become as fluent as a pharmacist in drug names. He keeps his current supply and their refills organized with a dogged precision.

"I need the Cipro and the Diflucan."

"Cleocin?"

"No. I have enough."

"AZT?"

"I stopped taking it last month, remember? Because of the white blood cells."

"Sure enough." Protocol 117 ended a while ago, DDI was licensed and released for general use, and Mr.

Soto has been taking alternating courses of AZT and DDI since.

He takes a total of seventeen different medications: fourteen by mouth, one injected under the skin, and two inhaled into the nose. Six are to be taken once a day, three are twice a day, two are three times a day, one is four times a day, two are every four hours while awake, one is before sleep. The others can be used as needed.

I asked him two weeks ago what he did all day. "I wait!" he said. We both began to laugh.

In any other language that might have meant many things. In our concrete vernacular, it means only one. Mr. Soto spends his days waiting for the right time to take each medication, exactly as prescribed.

March 1989
February 1990
October 1990
May 1992
August 1992
December 1992
May 1993

June 1993

His cough won't go away. I have tried all my old tricks, but nothing helps—not changing his antibiotics, or treating him for a sinus infection, or treating him for asthma, or for PCP, or convincing him to trade in his Marlboros for Carltons for a week. He coughs in the corridor and in the examining room, during meals and through the night. I can change the color of his sputum from green to white to green again with different antibiotic regimens, but still Mr. Soto coughs, the left side of his abdomen cradled protectively with one hand, a tissue held apologetically to his mouth with the other.

His chest X ray, that map of old battlegrounds, is too cluttered with the skeletons of old infections to reveal the footprints of a new one. His days of mild, easily treated pneumonias are gone. From the specimens of his sputum I send to the laboratory strange microorganisms now grow, bacteria and soil-dwelling fungi with multisyllabic names. Textbooks call them nonpathogens, meaning that they almost never cause human infections. An infection from a nonpathogen is like an infection from a mushroom spore, or a parsley seed, or a milkweed fluff. It means that some basic law of nature has broken down: an organism that usually grows in soil is rooting and growing in human tissue, all rules of nurture and habitat awry.

Journals now report more and more AIDS patients developing infections from nonpathogens. It would still be a big leap of faith for me to decide that Mr. Soto had an infection from one of the organisms the lab keeps isolating from his sputum. Even if I did, I would have a hard time treating him: most of these nonpathogens laugh at standard antibiotics; they drink them for breakfast and beg for more. For most of them the only available treatments are as toxic as the disease. Much better to keep looking for something in those lungs that I can do something constructive about.

Other than the cough, Mr. Soto is a miracle of finely tuned medication. His weight has been stable, his color good, his spirits high ever since the social worker stopped pestering him about his resuscitation and health proxy forms ("I'm still thinking"). Melissa, newly graduated from fourth grade, is now as tall as her tiny mother. When I headed into clinic today, mother and daughter were whispering together on their bench in the corridor. They both nodded to me, wary and silent. Mr. Soto had already been taken into one of the nurses' check-in rooms. As I passed by its closed door, I could hear him hacking apologetically around the thermometer held loosely between his back teeth. I no longer pay much attention to the oral temperatures the nurses record for him; I feel his forehead instead.

When I sit down at my desk, Mary delivers his chart directly into my arms instead of placing it behind the others in the door rack. "You might want to see him first," she says.

"He has to go fishing?"

"No." She looks at me a little strangely. "Not exactly."

I look down at the chart. She has written that his weight has dropped by seven pounds since last week. His oral temperature, even in its cough-aerated version, is 103°. She wasn't able to find his blood pressure to measure it. He has told her that he has been unable to swallow solids or liquids for days.

"How does he look?"

She shakes her head and vanishes without answering. When he appears at my door, Mary is supporting him by one arm, Mrs. Soto by the other.

I don't have to go through the usual ritual, or in fact any ritual at all. He is a collection of diagnoses held together with pills. If he can't swallow his pills he will fall apart, diagnosis by diagnosis. In the hospital, intravenous fluids and medications may function as some kind of temporary cement. His mouth is coated with thrush, despite his daily Diflucan, and a strain of candida resistant to Diflucan is almost certainly cascading down his esophagus, abrading its lining, turning every swallow into a sword. He needs one more medication, one more card on a balanced tower.

"Only for a few days, right?" he says thickly from the stretcher we have ordered to bring him down to the emergency room. He coughs, chokes a little. Mrs. Soto puts another pillow under his head, murmurs something in Spanish. The stretcher heads off down the corridor, mother pushing, daughter pulling, orderly walking alongside.

March 1989
February 1990
October 1990
May 1992
August 1992
December 1992
May 1993
June 1993

July 1993

I see Mr. Soto every day in the hospital, and every day he tells me he's feeling better. At first he looks impossibly ill lying against pillows in a hospital gown, but after a few days he actually does begin to look better. When I come to see him on the afternoon of his fifth day in the hospital his bedside chart shows that he hasn't had a fever in twenty-four hours. His bed is empty, though, and he himself is nowhere to be found.

At the far end of the ward corridor I can make out a familiar figure. Mrs. Soto has appropriated the bench under the window outside his room, as firmly as she ever tenanted her bench in the clinic. She gets to the hospital at 6:30 in the morning, the nurses tell me, and leaves at 9 or 10 at night. Sometimes she helps with his nursing. Sometimes she just sits and waits. When I come up to her she nods and beams. I nod and beam back. We have been nodding and beaming at each other for four years now, her English having apparently made as little progress as my Spanish. Mr. Soto has always been around for any actual communication between us. This is the first time, strangely enough, we have been left on our own.

I walk down the corridor to her bench."His fe-ver is gone!" I say slowly, enunciating. "That's good! Bueno! Do you know where he is? Donde—?"

"They have taken him downstairs for another chest X ray. They are concerned because although the fever has left, he coughs up some blood," she says matter-of-factly. In five years I have never heard her speak an English sentence.

"I thought you didn't speak English!"

She shakes her head, smiling. "My English. Is not good enough to speak. Usually I don't like, but now I have to speak, for him."

A strange way to put it, I think. I wonder what she means.

"Well, that's great. And it looks like he's getting better. He'll be home soon."

No answer. She is looking past me down the hall. "He is here."

The orderly deposits Mr. Soto's wheelchair next to the bench. He is rosy and grinning. "Much better! Just a little cough, now. No fever. I ate lunch!"

"You'll be home soon."

"I think so!" He glances over at Mrs. Soto. "My wife, she keep worrying I won't go home. But I know, I'll be home soon! The fever is gone."

The next afternoon his temperature chart has a spike in it like an Alp. He was almost 106° the night before. And from that day on he is feverish every night, huge spiking fevers that leave no room for misinterpretation. The wispy patches on his X ray spread and fuse into a massive pneumonia. His weight plummets. He is in the thick of something. We don't know what it is.

It could be anything, from an ordinary case of PCP to a pneumonia caused by one of those nonpathogens that have been crawling around his sputum for a month now. The only way to find out is to do a biopsy of his lung, a risky and uncomfortable procedure that we often try to circumvent by simply administrating treatment for all possible alternatives. In Mr. Soto's case, though, this kind of empiric treatment is impossible. He is too sick. He is allergic to too many things. Late one afternoon while I am in the clinic his resident explains the options to him and, surprised, calls me to report that Mr. Soto wants a lung biopsy and she has called the pulmonary specialists to consider him for one.

All that night I worry about Mr. Soto and his lung biopsy. I have had too many arguments with the pulmonary specialists about biopsies in the past to stop thinking about it. They are very choosy about the people whose lungs they biopsy. They don't want to do the procedure unnecessarily. They don't want to cause complications. Some people they decide aren't sick enough to warrant it. Some people they decide are too sick to weather it. I'm sure they're going to decide Mr. Soto is too sick, is too terminal, has exceeded his life expectancy by too many years. They'll never realize that he wants and deserves every last trick in the book, my tricks, their tricks, everyone's tricks. And then there's the compensation issue. Maybe they won't realize that he has Medicare and they'll be amply paid for their procedure. It's not supposed to matter to them, but it seems to make a difference sometimes.

By morning I've decided that if necessary I will write a letter to the president of the hospital and the chairman of the department to get Mr. Soto his biopsy. I'll go all out. I won't take no for an answer. I feel much better. I arrive at his bedside that afternoon planning my opening paragraphs. The room is quiet. Mr. Soto is snoozing, Mrs. Soto's chair by his side is empty. I can hear her moving around in his bathroom.

Mr. Soto stirs, opens an eye, closes it again. He's not usually this lethargic.

"Are you awake?"

He nods.

"We'll start working on getting you that biopsy right away."

He shakes his head. "I've had it."

"What?" He's had it? He's giving up?

His eyes stay closed. "I had it. They did it. This morning."

They did it? This morning? For a brief minute I am absolutely convinced he's hallucinating. They never do biopsies so quickly. They always argue, weigh the options, delay. But Mrs. Soto, coming out of the bathroom, nods and smiles.

"They did it," she says. "They said it went good. They will have the results after the weekend."

They did it. No letter to the president, the chairman, the board of trustees. I feel like I've run a marathon.

I call the pulmonary consultant for no good reason at all. I don't really have to thank him; this kind of thing isn't supposed to be regarded as a personal favor. But I can't help myself.

"You did it!"

"What a nice guy," says the pulmonary consultant. "We wanted to go all out for him." Mr. Soto evidently doesn't need my heavy hand to fight his battles.

Three days later, the results of the biopsy return. He has aspergillosis of the lung, a pneumonia caused by one of the nonpathogens in his sputum I have noticed and chosen to ignore. The news could be better, but it could be worse. It's a hard infection to treat successfully, mostly because Amphotericin, the best medication available for it, is a detergentlike compound that kills human cells almost as happily as it kills fungal cells, making it an extraordinarily toxic drug.

But Mr. Soto's endlessly unpredictable relationship with medications provides another surprise. He tolerates hefty doses of Amphotericin without a single side effect. His fever curve begins to blunt a little, the traced line on his bedside chart smoothing from Alps to foothills. He starts to eat again. His X ray stops getting worse, then begins to get a little better. The days drag on, every day a little better than the one before.

I go to see him one Friday before a three-day weekend. I have been coming into the hospital seven days a week now for six weeks, just to look in on him. Now I think I can slack off a little.

"Pretty good! Just a funny thing, my tongue feels funny. They think it's the new medicine."

He has been given a new pain reliever for the chest pain that has accompanied his pneumonia. And in fact his voice is a little different, a little thicker than usual. He sounds a little drunk. It probably is the new medicine. They've ordered it to be held and put him back on his usual Percocet. Everything else seems in order.

On Tuesday afternoon his room is darkened when I check back in. Mrs. Soto is sitting by the side of the bed. Mr. Soto is propped upright. When he sees me his face twists to one side. He gurgles, drools. Shrugs with one shoulder. I can't believe my eyes.

Over the weekend the right side of his face has become paralyzed and he has lost most of the strength in his right arm. The emergency CAT scan of the brain he had done on Saturday night showed an enormous mass displacing most of the tissue on the left side of his brain. The house staff has started him on medications for one of the common AIDS-associated brain infections.

He gesticulates wildly at me, screws up his face, looks at his wife for help. She now interprets for him as effortlessly as he ever did for her.

"He says that the dose of the Cleocin they are using is making him vomit like it used to do at home. I try to tell the residents but they don't listen. Maybe you can tell them?"

High-dose Cleocin always did make him vomit. I tell the residents. I also tell them, when they ask me what I think is going on in his brain, that the lemon-sized mass could be anything. An extension of his chronic sinus infections. Another focus of the aspergillus infection from his lungs. A tumor, one of the virtually untreatable brain lymphomas of very late stage AIDS. The only way to tell is a biopsy of the brain tissue itself, a gruesome procedure but relatively safe and painless. It will let us know what we're dealing with, although actually dealing with whatever it is will be something else altogether. The mass is so big, and Mr. Soto is so debilitated, that the residents think perhaps it's not worth it to find out. I suggest that we ask Mr. Soto. We all head together into his room. His resident sits on the edge of his bed and explains.

" . . . a little needle takes a piece of tissue to look at under the microscope. To see what it is. To give you the right kind of medicine. But, you know, it's probably going to be a kind of a hard thing to treat. Hard to help. Maybe you should think about it for a while."

Mr. Soto knows all about biopsies. He's already thought. He gesticulates wildly and unmistakably. He wants to know what it is and to get treated for it.

The resident goes to call the neurosurgeons. I listen to her on the phone for a few seconds before I head to the back of the nursing station for some forms. One more thing has to be taken care of. I take my turn on the edge of the bed.

"You remember a couple of years ago when we were talking about the machines? About, if you get really sick, whether or not you wanted to go on the machines? Remember how you were supposed to be thinking about it all this time?"

He gurgles unintelligibly, staring straight ahead. His left hand reaches swiftly out for my pen. His wife helps him move it across his Do Not Resuscitate forms. A big "Michael Soto" takes shape looping drunkenly all over the bottom of the page, banishing extraordinary measures and machines from his future. I can't think of anything else to say. I can't leave. We all three just sit there for a while.

Cynthia Wilson

APRIL 1991

"Pauline Wilson?"

With a sigh, the elderly black woman sitting in the waiting room gets to her feet and follows me into my room. Settled in my office chair, she drags her gaze from the opposite wall and lets it bounce briefly off my face. She has the resigned air of a subway rider who has taken

79

this particular trip many times before. She makes the tiniest motion with her head, her eyebrows go up a millimeter. This is my greeting, and it's all she can spare.

I've heard a little about Mrs. Wilson, but I've never met her before. When she has a problem she usually heads with the determination of a panzer tank for one of the doctors she already knows and trusts in the clinic. This week both members of this select group are on vacation. That Mrs. Wilson has allowed herself to be deflected to a stranger speaks loud for the urgency of whatever's bothering her.

Mrs. Wilson's chart is encyclopedic. Until last year it encompassed all the endemic problems of an inner city black woman except one. Now it's got them all.

She came from North Carolina to New York as a teenager and bore four children by three different men, all legal or de facto husbands for a shorter or longer period of time, none presently in the vicinity. She had regular housekeeping jobs until about ten years ago, when her health began to deteriorate. Now she is pushing sixty, overweight, diabetic; she has high blood pressure, asthma, arthritis, and occasional attacks of phlebitis. The usual cycling of the ages of man would have Mrs. Wilson winding down for a rest right about now. But, instead, on the jazzed-up carousel that is New York City, her life is beginning all over again.

One of Mrs. Wilson's sons went back to North Carolina as a teenager, and one son headed out to Brooklyn. Her daughters stayed with her in the Bronx.

Cynthia stayed sober, but Margie the baby went wild. First, Margie's five children arrived one after another at Mrs. Wilson's house for care and feeding while their mother was sent by the courts through yet another drug rehabilitation program. Then, about four years ago, Margie herself showed up on her mother's doorstep, emaciated and feverish. She died of AIDS eight months later. Her children, ages two through nine, stayed right where they were.

Mrs. Wilson began trudging the familiar patterns all over again: to the elementary school, to the pediatric clinic, to the Bureau of Child Welfare. To the food stamp office. To the school social workers, over and over again for Margie's wild little seven-year old. "He won't mind no one but me," Mrs. Wilson tells the social workers with a tinge of pride. Most of them write this down verbatim in their notes.

Last year, Mrs. Wilson got a phone call from an old friend, a man who had drifted in and out of her life in the early 1980s. He didn't exactly say why he was calling, only that he had been sick and wondered about her. It didn't take Mrs. Wilson long to put two and two together. When her own HIV test returned positive a month later she wasn't a bit surprised.

So now she comes to our clinic, sits on the bench where Margie used to sit, watches the traffic in the waiting room with unreadable eyes. Chronologically, she is by no means the oldest person we take care of—we have men and women in their late sixties and a few in their seventies—but when Mrs. Wilson hoists herself to her swollen feet to chase after the frenzied little boy who sometimes accompanies her, she is the oldest person in the world.

Today she is alone, slumped silently in the chair by my desk, waiting, I imagine, for the usual routine to begin. She's been in and out of the hospital so many times, been seen in so many hectic, disjointed clinics, been examined by so many doctors, nurses, social workers, and their trainees ("Go in and talk to Mrs. Wilson— she's a classic case") that she could probably write a script for me herself:

"Hello, Mrs. Wilson. I'm a doctor you've never seen before. I have all five volumes of your chart in front of me, but I still intend to obtain a complete history from you by asking you a series of extremely detailed personal questions. It's very important that you follow along. Now, let's see. What diseases do you have? What medicines do you take? Are you sure you take all those? You miss doses, I bet. Don't you? I thought so. Did you ever use intravenous drugs? Are you sure? Absolutely sure? Tell me about your past sexual partners. Ever had syphilis? Are you sure? We'll get to your leg pain in a second."

I decide to skip the preliminaries.

"What's up, Mrs. Wilson?"

She stares at the wall. "Ain't you gonna ask me my medical history?"

"Not unless you feel like telling it."

"It's all in the book."

That it is, reiterated over and over. Although Mrs. Wilson is asymptomatic from her HIV infection, all her other diseases are active and more than active. She is a regular at the chest clinic, the diabetes clinic, the cardiology clinic, and the medical clinic. Lately, though, she seems to be coming more and more often just to us. Maybe this is because, ironically, no one in our clinic appears to have taken much of an interest in her sex life. Instead, we have been occupied with her blood sugar (ranging from high to dangerously high), her asthma (on a hair trigger since her grandson adopted a cat), and her phlebitis ("No one to chase after them children but me").

Complete silence ensues. Maybe I shouldn't have ignored the usual formalities.

"Are you feeling bad today?"

She snorts, smiles a little at the wall. "Honey, I feel bad every day."

She keeps staring at the wall. Under her chair her feet have quietly begun to nudge each other, gently easing off her shoes. The cheap plastic moccasins, white with molded soles and imitation Navajo decorations in colored lanyard, have notched angry grooves into the puffy insteps. Freed, her toes neatly align the shoes into pair formation.

"Is it your leg?"

"My leg ain't so bad today, somehow."

"Is it your breathing?"

"That cat run away. My grandson, he be home looking for it right now."

Silence.

"So it sounds like you feel OK today?"

"I guess."

Silence.

"So what's up, Mrs. Wilson?"

"Nothin', I guess."

Silence.

"Dr. Marley, is she coming back soon?"

Only her toes, clenched over the railings of the chair, stop me from giving her a piece of my mind. Even so, my goodwill is disappearing fast.

"Mrs. Wilson, you can talk to me now, or you can wait two weeks for her to come back from vacation. It's your choice. Take your pick."

Silence.

"Come on, Mrs. Wilson. Have a heart. I have another six patients waiting out there."

Another snort. Under her chair the swollen feet begin feeling around for the shoes. She reaches down and jams each shoe over a foot, hooks the heels into place. Her face shows nothing.

"If I bring in my daughter, you all take a look at her?"

Of course. It would have to be something like that. But I must have missed something in my reading of the chart. One daughter with AIDS, dead. One daughter without, alive, healthy, two children of her own.

"Your daughter?"

"My Cynthia. She don't look too good to me. She got the thrush real bad. She can't eat, can't drink. Just stays in bed."

"I'm sorry, Mrs. Wilson. I didn't realize your daughter was still alive."

Suddenly she's standing. The flesh of her ankles spills out over the stiff white shoes. "That one's dead. This is the other one. She tell me and she tell me that she's fine but I know what I see. Cynthia got two kids of her own. Got all seven of them with me now. They all out looking for that cat. My luck, they find it."

Suddenly she's moving quickly, out the door. I reach out a hand to stop her, but she's gone.

April 1991

June 1991

"My mother told me you weren't going to ask no questions like that."

Cynthia Wilson is slumped so low in the chair that she is almost horizontal. She mutters something else I can't catch, then subsides. Her eyes close. As far as she is concerned, our interview is over.

This is Pauline Wilson's daughter, the late Margie's sister. Three weeks ago her mother shook her out of bed, dressed her, called a cab, and half-dragged, half-carried her into the clinic building and up to our fourth-floor walk-in clinic. There Cynthia opened her mouth a crack for the nurse to look in and sullenly signed her name to an HIV-test consent form. Her test was purely a formality. The exuberant candida infection the nurse saw in Cynthia's mouth, swirling patches of white on her palate and gums and down the back of her throat, spoke for itself. Two weeks later she was told the results of her test and given an appointment with me. Now she is here, her mother outside in the waiting room, holding Cynthia's coat and bag. Were it not for this praetorian guard, I'm sure Cynthia would have bolted hours ago.

I should have had the sense to avoid the whole topic of the source of her HIV infection. Gentle as I tried to be, it wasn't gentle enough for Cynthia, who is now curled up on the hard plastic seat with her back to me. Her mother has already told us that Cynthia has no idea how she got her infection. She's not a drug user, but many of her past boyfriends were. It was probably one of them that has turned her into a "no identified risk" case of AIDS, the category assigned by the Department of Health when the specific heterosexual who has shared his infection with a new case is unknown.

The moment Cynthia opened her mouth last month and let the nurse down the hall glimpse the back of her throat, she skipped over all the intermediate stages of HIV infection directly to the last one, AIDS. Anyone with an immune system so depleted that candida can luxuriate far down the throat, and with no other good reason for the immune depletion, has AIDS until proved otherwise. This kind of clinical reasoning allowed AIDS to be diagnosed in the early 1980s even though HIV hadn't yet been discovered. And in fact Cynthia is exactly the kind of AIDS case that we used to see during the first years of the epidemic, before HIV testing was possible. People who hadn't seen a doctor in years suddenly showed up with the most devastating manifestations of immune deficiency that hit like a bolt from the blue—one day they were trading on the stock exchange, hustling in the street, cooking in the kitchen; a week later they were at death's door. With HIV testing the disease seems elongated, spanning decades instead of months, but, of course, it's all an illusion. The book has always been the same length, but now we open it earlier and earlier and have to read more of the story. In the past, we could read only the last chapter, the denouement.

Cynthia's head is bent away from me into her chest. Her hair is downy, thinning, bronzed at the ends, black near the roots. I think idly that if she has stopped speaking to me permanently I can gauge when she started feeling bad by the length of her undyed roots. If hair grows at half an inch a month, it looks like she ran out of energy about three months ago.

It may be just as well that Cynthia has weathered the longest and possibly the worst piece of an HIV infection unconsciously, never aware of the sword hanging over her head. Could she have endured a prolonged wait for the almost inevitable? She has only to remember her sister to conjugate the future tense of her disease. When they had tried to "post-test counsel" her in the walk-in clinic about the meaning of her positive HIV test, she left the room.

I myself have no intention of forcing HIV counseling down the very sore throat of someone who is imitating a dying pigeon on my chair.

"So, Cynthia, what about your throat? Is it any better?"

Silence.

"Did the pill they gave you in the walk-in clinic make your throat any better?"

A murmur sounds very much like, "Can't swallow no pills."

This is very bad news.

"You didn't take the pills?" I try to cloak my dismay but it comes through nonetheless, nicking a hole in Cynthia's armor. She flings herself around, churning out all the past weeks' accumulated anger.

"What is WRONG with you all?" Her face is bright red, the variegated wisps of her hair spiking out around it. Her eyes are framed in black circles. Her mother thinks she has lost something like forty pounds in the last few months. She is now actually close to the ideal weight for her height, but something in the loose droop of her sallow cheeks makes her look much thinner. Flecks of white appear at the corners of her mouth. She spits out every word like a bullet.

"No, I didn't take them stupid pills. I told them stupids I couldn't eat nothing, I can't swallow nothing, not food, not pills, nothing. What they give me pills for when I tell them I CAN'T SWALLOW NOTHING?"

We stare at each other. The whites of her eyes glisten against her flushed face. I'm sure that if she had any strength she would be throttling me senseless, one too many cold, white-coated judgmental strangers in her exploding life. I'm thinking as fast as I can and I can think of nothing, absolutely nothing to reply except for the exact unvarnished truth.

"Then you have to come into the hospital."

I brace myself for another explosion, but none comes. Instead, Cynthia relaxes against the back of the chair, still staring at me, breathing fast but her high color fading. "When do I come in?"

"Right now, if you can."

She nods. "I guess I surely can." Her face has slackened into a weird peace, almost a smile. Now I'm the one showing the whites of my eyes. Something is wrong here. No one wants to come into the hospital. We tend to distort every rule of medical care to keep our patients out of the hospital, where the AIDS ward, despite endless well-meaning modifications, remains a slightly fetid reminder of everything they are trying to forget. We have all grown accustomed to constructing careful procrastinations ("Remember, if the fever goes on past Tuesday, you have to come in"), issuing impossible instructions ("Can you, say, drink a quart of water every three hours and then come back tomorrow and we'll see if your blood pressure has come up?"), and generally mangling ordinary clinical practice for a good cause. Ordinarily I would have cheerfully embarked along one of these routes with Cynthia ("Can you crush the pills up in apple sauce and get them down? We'll give it through the weekend . . ."), but evidently this particular compromise is not to be.

"You can come into the hospital for intravenous?"

"I guess." She still looks peaceful, almost beatific. She has probably misunderstood.

"For intravenous into the veins? With needles? In the hospital?"

Cynthia fixes me with her mother's impassive stare. She no longer looks like a madwoman in opera makeup; now she looks like exactly what she is, a thirty-five-year survivor of the Bronx at its worst.

"I know what them words mean, Miss. My older daughter she be acting up something fierce. She due next month but that don't stop her, the boys they be outside walking back and forth, back and forth all night they be calling her name, and then she go down to tell them scat, she don't come back. Then my other daughter she get scared in the bed alone, then boom she be in my bed too. I scream and scream but it don't matter, them girls they don't listen. They don't neither of them care about me. I tell them both they be sorry when I gone and now they can see just what it's like, they can go back with my mother, I can get me a little rest, is what I need, I can get me a rest."

She beams a smile my way.

April 1991
June 1991

September 1991

"So tell me what you had to eat yesterday."

Cynthia Wilson grins widely and settles back in her chair. I find myself grinning too. I actually don't care much about the vitamin and calorie counts I pretend to tally up these days. I just love watching Cynthia enjoy her food.

"Well, yesterday being Sunday, first I had some farina for breakfast. Then after church I had me some fried chicken, greens, mashed potatoes for lunch. Then in the afternoon I had me some popcorn and some pizza . . ."

Cynthia's pilgrimage through the land of the malnourished ended about two weeks ago when she woke up and realized that for the first time in more than six months she could swallow without pain. When I put her in the hospital last spring, the candida infection in her mouth and throat was easily treated, but even after it disappeared she still couldn't swallow. It didn't take the residents caring for her long to find the ragged sore at the bottom of her throat near her stomach that was making every bite an agony. For weeks afterward, though, she languished on the ward while the ulcer resisted all efforts at diagnosis and treatment. Actually, it was Cynthia herself who resisted most of the efforts; she took an instant dislike to each and every one of the specialists who were called in on her case and waved their biopsies and X rays away. But the tests that did get done were all negative: none of the usual bacteria or viruses seemed to be causing this ulcer, and none of the usual treatments took it away.

Three weeks of hospitalization left Cynthia no better than before, miserably sipping vitamin-fortified milkshakes, her two daughters sitting by her bed. Ebony, ten, cried and held her mother's hand. Charmain, fifteen, eight months' pregnant, sat glumly apart, obviously counting the seconds until she could leave. Then Pauline Wilson's phlebitis acted up. I came to visit Cynthia on the ward one day and found her dressed and ready to leave, scribbling her signature on the Against Medical Advice form her intern held. "My mother, she's in the Emergency," Cynthia said. "They say she gotta come in for blood clots in the lungs." She took a can of Ensure from the bedside table and stuffed it into her pocket. I didn't bother to volunteer the usual protests. At last count Pauline Wilson had seven children in her home, including Cynthia's two. If Pauline had to come into the hospital, Cynthia had to come out. The next morning Pauline had actually been admitted to Cynthia's recently vacated bed on the ward, while Cynthia was sipping Ensure at her mother's kitchen table.

Dragging herself into the clinic a few weeks after she left the hospital, Cynthia sat in my chair and stared at the wall. She was as silent as ever but no longer hostile, evidently having passed into some other stage of grief since her first angry visit. She stared at the wall while I read through every detail of her inpatient stay in a chart grown two inches thick in a month. Then I reached for my pad and wrote her a prescription for prednisone.

Steroid hormones, of which prednisone is one of the most frequently prescribed, have no logical place in the treatment of HIV infection. Steroids work their miracles by suppressing the body's immune response to whatever is bothering it, whether tumor, toxin, or microbe. While they effectively abolish all kinds of discomfort, from the itch of poison ivy to the pain of rheumatoid

arthritis, they do so at the expense of a generally damp-
ened immune system. When the discomfort steroids
soothe is caused by an infection, they mean trouble. The
reactions they suppress are the very barriers the body con-
structs against the infection's progress. HIV by itself pretty much gives infections carte blanche to proceed as they
will. No one really wants to smooth their way any further
with steroids.

But for some conditions there are simply no other
options. It looked very much like Cynthia had one of
them. Her giant esophageal ulcer seemed to contain no
microbes at all: it was simply the sign of an immune system crazed by HIV, a cyclone of psychotic cells unleashed
from all their usual restraints, drilling a hole into her tis-
sues for no good reason at all. Occasionally these cells
can be knocked back to their senses with AZT, but in
Cynthia's case AZT hadn't done the trick. The only other
option I could think of was prednisone, that major tranquilizer for hyperactive cells. A few weeks of prednisone
wouldn't do her immune system any lasting harm, although a longer course of the drug would be more dangerous.

"This is going to work," I told her. She rolled her
eyes.

But now, a month later, she's a different person.
She has gained back fifteen of her lost pounds in the
last two weeks. Her face is fuller, her scraggly hair
now evenly bronzed. Although she moved out of her
mother's apartment back into her own when fifteen-
year-old Charmain made her a grandmother two weeks

ago, Cynthia actually looks rested and serene as she finishes up with Sunday's menu.

"And then my daughter grilled some cheeseburgers. That was dinner. Then I had me my can of Ensure for dessert."

"Ensure?" Ensure is fine as food substitutes go, particularly if served chilled on ice to knock out some of that earthy vitamin taste. Even its manufacturers have probably never used it to cap off a lavish meal, however. I wasn't sure I knew Cynthia well enough to say what came to mind, but she said it for me, almost cackling with delight:

"'Cept for my baby's formula it was the only thing left in the house."

April 1991
June 1991
September 1991

May 1992

Cynthia is spilling over the seat of her chair, her thighs massive in orange Lycra, her belly a dome of dimpled folds under her halter top. A can of Ensure is clutched in her hand because once again, hard as it may be to believe, she is starving to death. I have done this to her myself, cutting off her food supply as firmly and cruelly as a trade embargo. I had to do it, and now I have to fix her up, but I'm damned if I know how.

Prednisone was Cynthia's miracle drug. Three pills a day smoothed over the hole in her esophagus almost overnight, and a little ordinary food turned her into a different person. Like one of those dehydrated sponge toys plunged into a glass of water, she flowered out into the most unexpectedly large and exotic creature. She had charm, she had energy. She took care of her infant granddaughter and her teenage daughters and her mother and her nieces and nephews. She cooked, she cleaned. She shopped. She pierced her nose. She took a part-time job selling hot dogs from a cart on her corner. She knew she had AIDS, but it didn't daunt her anymore; she had, after all, risen from the brink of the grave. She felt better with AIDS than she had felt six months before without it. She began doing a little comparison shopping in sofas and washing machines.

After three months, though, the miracle had become a little too miraculous. Cynthia was becoming bigger and bigger; she had passed the 200-pound mark and showed no signs of stopping. She was flushed, florid, her cheeks glowing with sweat as she huffed her way in and out of the clinic, pushing her baby granddaughter in a stroller, a hot dog in her hand. Her hair began to thin; her blood sugar, tested monthly, rose from normal to a little high to a frankly diabetic range. She was becoming a steroid monster.

"Time to stop the prednisone," I told her months ago. "Just taper it down a little at a time. Here—I'll write you out a schedule. You'll get down to 10 milligrams a day by the end of the week, and then we'll change the size of your pills to 2.5 milligrams and go down very slowly." She couldn't stop taking the pills all at once: we had to taper them slowly down so that her own adrenal glands would get reaccustomed to manufacturing the low levels of steroids she needed to survive. I wrote out a detailed schedule. She nodded, asked intelligent questions, put the schedule in her handbag, and didn't follow it.

"I thought my throat started hurting a little that day I went down to 7.5, so I took another 20," she would report. "Just to be safe."

I tried to scare her with stories of what happened to people who took steroids: ". . . terrible infections, your bones get weak, you'll have to take insulin like your mother, your skin gets thin and striped red and white . . ." It turns out that it's very difficult to scare someone newly returned from the brink of the grave. But what did scare her were those twinges of pain she felt in her throat whenever the prednisone dose got too low.

When her chest X ray showed an abnormality, I began to panic. That was what I had been fearing all along, something like this little unassuming nodule in the right lung, possibly nothing, possibly the beginning of a bad infection. I stared at it in the darkness of the radiology view room and realized the time had come for desperate measures.

I demanded that Cynthia bring in all her medications and unceremoniously tossed her stash of 10- and 20-milligram prednisone pills into the trash. I issued her enough 2.5-milligram pills for a week of the taper schedule I wanted her to follow. From now on she would come to the clinic once a week for a week's supply of pills, which would steadily decrease in number until she could come off them completely.

For three weeks I congratulated myself on my resourcefulness. Then came the day Pauline Wilson stopped in the clinic, motioned me out into the corridor, and held up an empty bottle of prednisone. "I knew there's a reason she be stopping over to see me all the time," said Mrs. Wilson. Her own asthma frequently became so bad that she needed to take prednisone for short periods of time, and she had accumulated a store of remnant pills in her medicine cabinet. Over three weeks Cynthia had helped herself to them all.

I sent Cynthia for another X ray: the nodule had grown a little. I hung up all her X rays for her to see, and she looked appropriately grave. I showed her the insulin needle she would have to start using if she clocked in another blood sugar result above 500. I told her I wanted her to be taking one 2.5-milligram prednisone pill every other day by the end of the following week, because that would be the day I would stop writing her prednisone prescriptions. I promised her that if the hole in her throat came back I would find another, better way to fix it up.

She did exactly what I told her to do. She stopped taking her prednisone by the end of the following week, and the reason I can be so sure of this is that, two weeks later, she is here in my office, massive, weeping in pain and frustration, in her hand no longer a hot dog but a can of Ensure. Still huge, still rosy, she has lost almost fifteen pounds in the space of fourteen days. The hole in her throat has come back with a vengeance. Even the Ensure barely goes down. Between sniffles she spits into a plastic cup so as not to have to swallow even her saliva.

She doesn't have to say anything, and neither do I. I know she's frightened, and she knows I'm sorry. We both know I've made a promise I'm not sure I can keep.

> *April 1991*
> *June 1991*
> *September 1991*
> *May 1992*

June 1992

"You know that drug called thalidomide?"

Cynthia, lounging on the chair, shrugs and shakes her head. For once, I'm glad of her droop. What I was fearing was the kind of reaction I myself have to that name, with its connotations of the forbidden and monstrous. But thalidomide hasn't made it into Cynthia's lexicon; not even when I prod her can she summon it to mind.

After the wave of birth defects thalidomide caused when it was sold as a tranquilizer in Europe in the 1960s, the drug has formally been unavailable in the United States. But of course, like most other banned and dangerous substances, this one turns out to be quite marvelous in its own way and also relatively easy to obtain. In Europe and Australia it has shown excellent results in the treatment of throat ulcers like Cynthia's. And after only a few phone calls I have managed to find a domestic source for thalidomide, the national Hansen's disease center in Carville, Louisiana. There it is distributed under the most stringent and restricted circumstances for the treatment of leprosy and of ulcers like Cynthia's that are refractory to all other agents.

"So that's the drug it looks like you need. It has almost no side effects. It might make you a little drowsy. You just have to make absolutely sure you don't get pregnant while you're taking it."

This is actually a slight oversimplification on my part. The Food and Drug Administration in Washington, D.C., whose blessing Cynthia and I need before the Carville laboratory will send me a shipment of the drug, is less than enthusiastic about my plans. Or, at least, the first FDA administrator I spoke to on the phone yesterday seemed quite adamant. "Oh, no, Doctor, I don't think we can release it to you," she had said emphatically. "We're very concerned about anyone giving it to a woman of childbearing potential."

The clerk's supervisor, my next phone call, grudgingly admitted that Cynthia was an ideal candidate for the drug but warned me that the agency would be taking an active interest in Cynthia's sex life and her means of birth control for the duration of her treatment. Although they haven't yet sent me the supply of paperwork, I am expecting the worst. To be completed monthly, in duplicate. No form, no drug.

As well as I've come to know Cynthia over the past year, it hasn't been well enough to overcome her intense dislike of personal questions, especially when she's feeling sick. She responds to all the routine queries regarding sex, condoms, and birth control with sullen silences and abrupt departures. The telephone service in her apartment has just been shut off for failure to pay an outstanding long-distance bill. Now when she heads out of the clinic she's gone until she comes back; even her mother can't always get in touch with her for us.

"So you're going to have to, uh, keep me up to date on your period and your, uh, sex life and all of that. OK?"

She doesn't raise her head or answer.

"You really have to make sure that you don't get pregnant. OK? Is that all right with you?"

"Hooo-eee!"

I'm prepared for every form of sullen disapproval from Cynthia, but what I'm not prepared for are the guffaws of laughter that are now bubbling out of her. My injunction that she not get pregnant is clearly the funniest thing she has heard in some time. I can almost hear her jaws creak as they part painfully to let the giggles out. She wipes her eyes and spits into the saliva cup that is now her constant companion.

"Pregnant! Ain't much chance of that. The government don't want me to get pregnant, well you can tell them that I don't want to get pregnant even more. I don't want them kids I got. I tell you, I do it all over again, I wouldn't have either one of them girls. My daughter she ain't learned nothing from that baby, she out all the time now, the baby be hollering, she go out to get Pampers she don't come back. I tell her I feel sick to fix me something to eat you know what she do? She make steak. She knows I can't eat no steak. I go to sleep, I wake up, there's a piece of black steak next to me. And she's gone. So I go to bed hungry. Can't she see what I look like? Ain't she got eyes in her face?

"What I want is my own place. Just for me and the baby. That's my baby now. I took care of that baby since the day it was born. My daughter she may be that baby's mother, but she ain't no mother. That baby don't have no mother. Them other two, they'll see what it's like without a mother someday. You can go tell these government people that I ain't going to get pregnant that's for damn sure."

She fixes me with a penetrating eye. A strange amalgam of health and disease, my massive starving Cynthia, her diminishing flesh hanging looser and looser, flopping in garish Lycra casings, her complexion still steroid-ruddy with ashy gray overtones, a white crust of dried Ensure on her cheek. I wish very much that I could package her at this moment and send her entire to the FDA, optimally COD to that most officious administrator who doubted I would be able to obtain thalidomide for a woman of childbearing age and potential. No matter how copious and detailed the paperwork they're planning to send me, and how many duplicates they're going to require, it's going to be hard to capture Cynthia's views of pregnancy with any kind of accuracy on a form.

April 1991
June 1991
September 1991
May 1992
June 1992

December 1992

I haven't seen Cynthia in almost three weeks, and it looks like I'm not going to be seeing her today either. Her appointment was an hour ago, but when I scan the waiting room she's nowhere in sight, nor are any of her trappings: no teenage daughters lounging sullenly in corners, no gaily colored carriage in which her granddaughter rides.

It is almost six months ago now that a small cardboard box arrived on my desk express mail from Carville, Louisiana, containing sixty white, anonymous-looking, 100-milligram thalidomide pills. I broke open the blister packs they were shipped in and repacked them into a spare pill vial, then lettered a reasonable facsimile of a standard medication label ("take one twice a day") and slipped the vial into the pocket of my lab coat, ready to hand over at Cynthia's next clinic appointment. Although I had never seen Cynthia's one-room apartment, I had the feeling that medication housed in anything but its usual amber plastic was unlikely to survive there long enough to be ingested per schedule.

I had looked forward to seeing thalidomide perform its miracles on Cynthia just the way prednisone had, transforming her from pain-ridden to painfree, thin to fat, limp to smiling over a week's time. I had figured without the FDA and its forms. Surly and starving before the paperwork even arrived, Cynthia slid so quickly downhill that I could barely get her to open her eyes and glance at the stack of information sheets and consent forms that finally reached my desk, let alone read and sign them. I had no choice but to put her back on prednisone. Within a week she was blooming again, rosy and beaming, signing her forms with a half-eaten tuna-fish sandwich balanced in foil on her lap.

Instead of creating a miracle, her thalidomide pills perpetuated one. They turned out to be the clean-up squad behind the parade, such sober, responsible pills next to that flashy, blowzy prednisone. Taking one thalidomide pill twice a day, Cynthia was able to taper down her prednisone over a week's time and—she said—never notice the difference. I made a point of asking with narrowed eyes about any remaining stashes of steroids, but she vigorously denied their existence. Her throat remained whole and functioning. She ate enough to gain some weight, but the bloated, balloon-float figure the steroids had molded began to deflate.

Three weeks ago all had seemed well. But where is she now? Her absences, unlike those of other patients, are impossible to interpret. She could be home because she feels too sick to move, or she could be out looking for a washing machine. Both circumstances have prompted prior truancies and, without a phone number to call, all we can do is wait. I have another supply of thalidomide in my pocket—Carville mails me a month's worth at a time. At some point soon I plan to stop the drug and see if she can last for a while without any medicine for her throat at all, but I'm not in any particular rush. It has been almost two years now that Cynthia has been bouncing between metabolic catastrophes. She needs a rest.

The phone on my desk shrills just as I am thinking that I wouldn't mind a small oasis myself in the windy wasteland of Cynthia's health. With her ups, her downs, and her thalidomide, she has been occupying great chunks of my time with worry and paperwork. But Mrs. Wilson's impassive voice on my telephone puts that dream on hold.

"I'm calling about Cynthia."

"Oh, hi, Mrs. Wilson. She's supposed to be here right now. Where is she, do you know?"

A mirthless laugh, one of Mrs. Wilson's specialties.

"She be there eventually, I guess. She told me she was gonna come. I told her she better after all she been up to."

My oasis on the horizon has shimmered into nothing. All I see is trouble, more trouble, with Cynthia, the person on the forbidden drug without a telephone. Now what?

"Mrs. Wilson, what has she been up to?"

"I just wanted to say, maybe you all want to check her for drugs, is all."

"Oh, no, Mrs. Wilson."

"She be lounging around here, can't walk straight, can't talk straight. Yesterday she fell down. Sunday I have my mother over here from Brooklyn and Cynthia goes in the living room with everyone there, just laughs and goes."

"Goes?"

"Goes. You know. She brings in a bucket, and she just go."

"She peed in your living room?"

"That's what I said. You all better check her out. She and her kids, all three of them all there in that room of hers by themselves, maybe she be thinking she back a kid now too. I just don't know."

"Mrs. Wilson, if she doesn't come in today, can you get her in here next week?"

Another laugh. "Ain't no one ever got Cynthia to a place she don't want to be."

Truer words were never spoken. But when I hang up the phone and look into the waiting room, there is Cynthia. I usher her right into my cubicle.

"So, uh, Cynthia, how are you?"

"All right."

She looks flushed and a little wild, doesn't meet my eyes.

"Is everything going all right?"

"Uh-huh."

"Your throat is OK? Are you taking your medicines?"

She lists them impeccably.

"Nothing's, uh, going on that I should know about?"

She shrugs, shakes her head, twists around to un-hook her jacket from the back of the chair.

"Wait a second. We're not done yet."

"Oh." She replaces her jacket, folds her hands in her lap, stares at me, exasperated.

"Your mother's a little concerned about you."

"How you know that?"

"She, uh, thinks you may not be feeling so well."

"How she know that? She tell me she don't want to see me round no more."

Was that before or after you peed in her living room? But I don't say it.

"She's still concerned about you."

Shrug.

"You're not using any, uh, drugs at all, are you?"

She looks at me, disgusted. "I don't do that stuff." Reaches back for her jacket again.

"Wait a second. How's your head doing?"

"What d'you mean?"

"Do you have a headache?"

Silence. Then, a little nod. A long shot pays off.

"It hurts a lot?"

She nods, looks as sheepish as she is capable of looking.

"Were you planning on mentioning that at all, by any chance?"

"Thought maybe it would go away."

"How long have you had it for?"

"Week."

"An entire week?"

"Week, two. Don't really matter."

"Does it ever go away?"

"Nah."

"How come you didn't tell me?"

Cynthia, no dope, just rolls her eyes at this one.

I reach for the phone, wondering which one of us was wishing for that oasis more. In Mrs. Wilson's world, strange behavior means drugs until proved otherwise. But what it means to me, in conjunction with Cynthia's headache and that flushed, slightly wild look of hers, is an infection in the brain or its coverings. Cynthia has just written herself another ticket into the hospital, and she knows it as well as I do.

"So you goin' to put me in?"

I nod. "You bet."

She drops her eyes, rubs her forehead with a hand. "It's OK. I better rest up some anyway. My daughter just tell me last night she due in June."

April 1991
June 1991
September 1991
May 1992
June 1992
December 1992

July 1993

Cynthia is sitting in the chair by my desk. For the first time in two years she looks all right. Neither flushed nor ashen. Neither bloated nor emaciated. Neither drooping nor manic. She looks at me calmly, the way a patient is supposed to look at a doctor. A new experience for the both of us.

She left the hospital in early spring after a long and extremely unsatisfactory stay. No one ever established any kind of a good explanation for her strange behavior of last winter. All we knew is that it went away. As best as they could determine in the hospital, it wasn't due to street drugs or to any of her medications. She had no infection in her brain. She didn't have a dementia due to HIV, which almost never gets better. The only thing we could find in Cynthia's case was a bad infection in one of her nasal sinuses. For lack of anything else to treat, we treated her for sinusitis, and everything got better. Her headaches vanished, her demeanor lost its strangeness. She smiled, she laughed. When it was time for her to leave she thanked everyone. She was a different person.

Finally, the green oasis. We have arrived.

"So! How are you doing?" I'm ready, more than ready for a brief, civilized session with her, full of idle pleasantries and reminiscence, with no untreatable complaints, insoluble problems, or disturbing phone calls. We both deserve it after this long acquaintance of ours that has been only a battle from first to last.

She gazes straight into my eyes.

"Not so good."

My jaw must be dragging in my lap.

"I don't believe it. You look so . . . great." This is not a response that would win me congratulations among the cognoscenti of the medical interview. I should be expressing nonjudgmental concern, but my viscera have spoken for me on this one.

"I mean, that is to say, I'm sorry to hear that. Is it your head? Your throat. . . ?"

"Nah." She shrugs. "I feel fine. But my damn nosy neighbors, they notified the Child Welfare on me. So now I gotta go back over to my place and see what's what. I been staying with my mother, and I guess my kids, they're both underage. My youngest daughter, she supposed to be staying with her godmother, but she come back home and the two of them are doing things they shouldn't be doing, having company and all. So I was supposed to go over there today but my mother tell them I have a doctor appointment, so I'll probably be going back tonight. My daughter she supposed to go talk to the Child Welfare lady about going into a group home. Since I can't control her. She say she want to go. They both want to go. But I say they don't know what those places is like."

This is one of the longest speeches I have ever heard out of Cynthia's mouth, and it's not over yet.

"What I really need is some sleeping pills. If you had given me some before when I ask you, I would have gone to sleep last night and never waked up. That house, I can't stand the noise, the baby she's at someplace where she's always carrying on. And the new baby, he never shut up. Just like his daddy. That boy he say it ain't his baby now, but you look at that noisy baby you know who he come from. I tell my daughter she better take him to court for that baby's papers right now. But she's almost eighteen and she's all developed and she got the kids but mentally she I don't know what. She a baby herself. She be playing spades with her friends till three, four in the morning and I be doing everything for this baby too. I buy the Pampers, I take care of him, she go spend the night at her friends'.

"Last weekend I went to my mother's house, and I just stayed. It's so quiet. The kids she got there is older. My house, I can't stand it. My mother and I, we talk, we watch TV. My mother say, that's my problem, I let them kids get to me. I got to take care of myself. She say I should stay with her for two, three months and rest up.

"I was real upset yesterday. My mother tell me my daughter having sex. My baby daughter. Ebony she tell my nephew and he tell my mother. She almost thirteen. She say we never talk but last night we had a long talk.

She didn't have much to say. I just tell it to her like it is. I tell her if I could do it again I ain't never would have had them kids. Never. When I go, I tell them, they'll see things different. They just been lucky so far. That Charmain, she'll be eighteen in November and I'm going to put the apartment in her name and I'm just going to go. Get me a one-bedroom. And when I go I take my baby with me. My Tamisha. She my baby, she a little devil and she get into everything but I don't think her mother take good care of her. She hit her too much. When I go, she go too."

Cynthia stops, waiting, I guess, for what I have to say. I have nothing to say. I have won a certain acclaim among my colleagues for fixing up Cynthia's esophagus, her diabetes, her who-knows-what-it-was crazies of last winter. I never stopped to think, and never thought to ask, how little I have fixed up Cynthia. For a few seconds I look at my lap, at the wall, anywhere except her calm eyes, looking at me the way a patient looks at a doctor, waiting for me to do something to make it better.

Eddie Rios

NOVEMBER 1989

"Have a seat, please. I'm Dr. Zuger." And sit as far away from me as you can—if I wind up catching the lice you undoubtedly have, I'm going to be very unhappy.

"Sir? Why don't you have a seat?" If I had any sense I'd put a pair of gloves on right this minute. I'm starting to itch already.

Eddie Rios can hear none of my silent thoughts, but he doesn't appear to hear the spoken ones either. He doesn't sit down. He paces, rapidly scratching a raw section of his left forearm, inspecting the examining room, the chairs, the table, the wall appliances. As he passes behind me I have the feeling he is inspecting my head. He coughs juicily. My scalp begins to crawl.

"Mr. Rios!"

I manage to break through: he looks at me and a great broad toothless grin splits his face.

"Sorry. They tell me alla time at the other. Make me wait in the. Drive 'em." He shakes his head and sits. He begins to drum the desk with his fingers, bobbing his head to the rhythm. His feet begin to tap in a different rhythm. He half rises from his chair, then catches my eye and sinks back down again. Begins to claw his other forearm. Meets my eyes. Tries to stop. Sits on his hands. Grins again.

"Pretty juiced up, aren't you?" Maybe this hyperactivity isn't caused by lice after all, but a more pharmacologic stimulus.

"Always like this. Can't sit. Haven't used. Kids back." He bobs his head enthusiastically. Another big grin. He doesn't seem to have a tooth in his head other than the big jagged one in the left front, but he bares the void without a hint of self-consciousness. His eyes are bright black marbles. I briefly try to estimate his pupil size with an eye to figuring out what is speeding him up like this, but the pupil is indistinguishable from the rest of the glossy globes. His hands pop out from under his legs, uncontrollable, and begin to play boogie on his corduroy knees. He shuts his eyes in ecstasy and jives.

Mr. Rios's methadone program has sent him here, the crumpled note he has placed on my desk says, for "management." They give no clue as to what is to be managed. So far it seems to be an itch, a cough, and a setting of 78 rpm in a 33⅓ rpm world. I wonder if he ever finishes his sentences.

"Mr. Rios!"

"Yes!" He jerks his eyes open, fixes them on me. His fingers flutter a little more boogie, then stop.

"Let's talk a little, OK?"

"OK! Yep, sure! You bet!"

"How long have you been coughing like that for?"

"Since I was. Hospital last. TB. Stopped taking."

I don't like the sound of this sequence, which resembles the cheerful song of a person with TB who stops taking his medication a few weeks after he begins to feel better and reverts into an aerosol can of infection. Half of me wants to back out the door to go fetch a mask for him, and one for me too. The other half wants to lean forward and grip him by the shoulders, shake slightly, and make him focus. Equally motivated forward and back, I move nowhere.

"Would it be possible for you to slow down a little so I can figure out what you're saying?"

Big grin, fading quickly as he makes a herculean effort to oblige.

"Always cough. Got pneumonia so many times I can't count. Hospital last. TB. Stopped taking."

Oh, God. "What?"

He tries again. "Went to the hospital last year. They say my X ray look like it was maybe TB. I drank medicines, then they say don't drink them no more."

"So it wasn't TB?"

"No. Skin test."

"You have a positive TB skin test?"

He nods, starts to drum again.

There. I have gathered a piece of information. At this rate we will grow old together.

"How long have you been HIV for? Very slowly."

"I got tested 1986. But I been sick long long before that. I shoulda got tested sooner cause my wife got it too. I think I shoulda got tested earlier so she didn't get it but thanks God she still OK. She never got sick. I got pneumonias, then last year they say it was the PCP."

We grin at each other. This is very good progress.

"Are you taking any medicines?"

"Gonna be honest. Bactrim, AZT."

"They told you to take those but you're not taking them." I'm beginning to catch on here.

"PCP both crazy drugs. Foster kids. Program. Kids back." When he found out he had AIDS he went crazy. Went back to using drugs. His wife too. They figured, what did it matter now? Their kids got taken away from them by the Child Welfare authorities and put in foster care. And then something made them come up for air.

They enrolled in a methadone program. They want to get the kids back. Now they have to convince the Bureau of Child Welfare that they are clean, domiciled, reconciled, and fit.

"Where are the kids?"

"Brooklyn. Visit. OK."

He nods emphatically. The kids have all escaped the family infection. "So it's important for you to stay clean, huh?"

"Told you. Always like this. Asthma kid. Scratch."

He was an asthmatic, eczema-ridden child. He always coughs. Always scratches. Only now do his cough and itch attract any attention. People think he has TB, think he has lice. In fact, he is just as always. With the possible addition of a little extra juice. The jury's definitely out on that one.

"You're really not using anymore?"

"Honest. No more. Kids back."

He begins to cough discreetly into one hand. The other scratches a weeping red patch behind his ear.

There are coughs and there are coughs. This is a cough with a capital C, heading up from deep down near his diaphragm, giving unmistakable evidence of something wet, sticky, and infected somewhere in those dark alveoli.

"I'm just going to pull on a pair of gloves here and listen to your chest, if you could lift your sweatshirt up for me . . ." His grin fades quickly. Maybe it's the gloves: no one likes to be examined by latex-covered hands. I usually don't wear gloves unless I am forced to protect myself from HIV-filled ooze—they make for an instant feeling of estrangement between examiner and examinee, hard feelings all around. But Mr. Rios is just too itchy. Call me picky, but any small crawling parties passing between us would make for even harder feelings.

Two hours later, his grin is gone completely. At least I assume it is—I can't really see behind the pink foam mask now obscuring most of his lower face. Outlined on the emergency chest X ray I sent him for after I heard a racket in his lungs is something that looks very much like TB. Masked and still gloved, I must be getting just as remote to him as he is becoming to me. For a first visit to the clinic, during which the experts encourage the forging of a bond between patient and health-care system, this one has not been a notable success.

"Telling you," he says disgustedly, muffled in layers of foam, "same thing before. It's not. Telling you, it's not."

His black button eyes are dull. He claws his right elbow with abandon. His feet tap time as he is loaded into the wheelchair that will take him down to the emergency room. There he will be deposited into the isolation room, the way station to one of the isolation beds in the hospital where all potential cases of TB are housed until their lack of contagion is proved. These beds are few and usually in demand. I have had patients waiting for days behind the closed door of the isolation room in Emergency for one of them to open up. Isolated patients tend to be forgotten about in the ER bustle, where the louder and more visible you are, the more attention you get. After a few days patients behind the isolation door begin to take on the desperate asthenic glaze of the longtime solitary confinee.

But there is absolutely nothing else I can do with this poor itchy man and his left upper lobe infiltrate.

"Sorry," I mutter as the orderly wheels him out of my office. Maybe it's not TB. But maybe it is. It beats me why I am apologizing for preserving the public health, even at the expense of an infectious toothless grin and shiny eyes.

November 1989
....
July 1990
....

"So how you been? You been OK?"

What was that? I ask a lot of people how they are in the course of a day. Almost nobody asks me first. I look up from the chart on my desk, a little ashamed that I barely remember this guy. A very high, very itchy person with a very mucky cough. Angry with me. As I read over my note of almost nine months ago I am surprised that he has come back, let alone that he is expressing any social concern for how I've been.

"Oh, er, just fine. Just fine. And yourself?"

"Good. Real good. Off the stuff. Getting my kids back. Gonna get some new teeth. See?" He bares his lips to reveal no teeth at all. "'Ulled all 'em." He leaps up to look at his bare gums in the mirror over the examining room sink. Leaps back into his chair to beam at me. Scratches enthusiastically at a large scaly patch behind his left ear. It's all coming back to me.

"Well! That's just great."

"Yeah. Can't wait to eat again, great!" Big toothless laugh. Right hand moves up to left ear, left hand drags it back. He firmly sits on both hands and laughs again. The laugh turns into a big juicy cough, which the hands fly out to cover, too late.

At least he is finishing most of his sentences now. Nothing much else seems to have changed. I wonder with something more than idle curiosity if he did turn out have TB after all. I went on vacation a few days after he was put in the hospital last fall, and on my return he had completely slipped my mind. It is unfortunate that I didn't keep closer track of him, since I'm not likely to find out too much about his hospital stay this afternoon. The clinic clerk has already told me that, as is frequently the case, his hospital chart is nowhere to be found. And he himself doesn't seem any more adept at narrative, let alone dialogue, than he was before.

"So how is your cough, Mr. Rios?"

"Listen, you gotta give me my medicines. I didn't get them all this time. My ADAP just come through last week. About time. No way I could pay for no medicines before. But those prescriptions they gave me, they're way out of date. So you gotta write more."

ADAP is the AIDS Drug Assistance Program, New York State's very generous medication insurance for HIV-infected state residents. The list of medications ADAP will subsidize is updated frequently and includes dozens of the most commonly prescribed medications for HIV-related conditions, ranging from vitamins to cutting-edge antibiotics with enormous price tags. For most of our patients, ADAP supplements the Medicaid coverage that funds most of their medical care and medications. For the few who don't have Medicaid, because they are still able to work, or because their assets exceed Medicaid stipulations, ADAP provides welcome relief from enormous medication bills—but only up to a point. Half paupers, half princes, these patients can afford without a thought the $12,000-a-year recombinant bone marrow growth factors that keep their HIV-depleted blood counts high and healthy, but when we write them a $15 prescription to decongest their noses from a non-HIV-related cold, or to treat their very ordinary hypertension, they sigh and shake their heads and ask if it can't wait till the first of the month.

Mr. Rios, when we last met, had evidently not been organized enough even to get himself an ADAP card and had been unable to pay for anything at all.

"You don't have Medicaid?"

His eyes widen. "Oh, now I do. Then, I had a problem. But I told you, everything's good now. So all you gotta do is write them slips, I won't be no more trouble."

Ordinarily a patient telling me what I gotta do rubs slightly against the grain, particularly when the instructions are repeated. I don't know why I'm not more irritated. Possibly I am becoming a saint.

"All right, OK, we'll get there. First you have to tell me what medicines you're supposed to be taking."

A great big shrug.

"You don't know what medicines they wanted you to take when you left the hospital?"

"Hey, that was a long time ago. I don't remember what they said, six, seven things, I don't know. Whatever you say is OK with me."

"Do you remember what they were treating you for in the hospital?"

Big laugh. "They wasn't treating me for nothing. They wasn't nothing me. They put me in that room, they don't even come check if I'm still alive."

Oh, no. This sounds like big trouble.

"So, uh, how long would you say you were actually in the hospital?"

He shrugs. "Couple of days."

People with X rays that looked like his don't receive honorable discharges from the wards after only a couple of days. Particularly not if nobody is treating them for nothing.

"You signed out, I guess."

"Yeah, well, like I said, they weren't treating me or nothing. So I told them I hadda go, and I did, I hadda go to court for the kids. So I said, OK, I'm gonna leave, get me the papers to go I'll sign. So they said, OK, you can sign, just take your medicine. So like I says, that's why you gotta write me the medicines."

A mist is starting to form before my eyes.

"Now just let me see if I've got this straight. Nine months ago I put you in the hospital because I thought you had TB. You stayed there for a couple of days, then you signed out. You told them just to give you TB pills and you would be sure to take them. But you somehow neglected to mention that you couldn't pay for the pills. So for the last nine months you've been going around coughing all over everybody you know, including your kids, I bet, and now you show up here and tell me you need your medicines? Is that right?"

My voice seems to getting a little higher, but I can't help it. He is scratching furiously again. Clearly, he knows he shouldn't like the sound of what he's done, but he can't really see the problem.

"So where have you *been* for the last nine months?"

"*Told* you, I been busy, real busy. I got offa everything, offa methadone, offa everything. I got my teeth pulled. I fixed up my Medicaid and my ADAP. Got an apartment. Got a phone. And now I'm here, OK? Anyway, like I told you, I always cough. Always. See?" He coughs. "This ain't nothing. But they said to me, I absolutely gotta take that medicine, and so that's why you gotta—"

I hold up my hand before he says it again. My saintly characteristics have vanished.

"Don't say it. Don't say anything. Don't move. Don't leave this room. And don't you cough either."

Ten minutes later, masked and escorted ("Don't let him out of your sight!"), he is on his way down to get another chest X ray. I sit and fume for a minute. I don't know who to be angrier at, this blithe Typhoid Mary who has just coughed in my face or the ward personnel who let him escape last fall to cough all over the city. They could have tried to hold him in the hospital against his will, a "health criminal," until they proved he wasn't contagious. They could have found a visiting nurse to give him his pills. They could have done many things, and they did none of them. I wish he hadn't coughed on me again.

Two hours later I am eating crow. I have called the TB laboratory, and it turns out that an assortment of Mr. Rios's blood, sputum, and urine specimens did manage to get cultured for TB last fall. All of them were signed out as definitely negative. I have looked at his chest X ray of today: it is crystal clear, only a thin scar in the part of the lung where that big juicy infection used to be.

As much as I hate to admit it, he is right: all I gotta do is write him his medicines. If what he had was in fact TB (possible even with the negative cultures), and we'll never know if it was or not, it healed itself. He needs medicine to ensure that it doesn't come back, and his family needs TB tests and chest X rays to make sure they haven't been infected. If what he had was actually something else, it looks like it's gone. Things do go away, every now and then, without benefit of antibiotics, Medicaid, or ADAP, although it certainly helps to have all these, not to mention an apartment, a telephone, and a set of teeth, when facing an HIV-infected future.

"All right, I guess you can take that mask off now." I can't be gracious about this: it is pure fluke of circumstance that this character has landed on his feet. He, however, seems to operate from a boundless natural courtesy. After he disentangles himself from the elastic bands holding the mask around his face he neither mutters nor coughs defiantly in my face. He doesn't say, "I told you so," or storm out of the room in a huff. Instead, he gives me a big toothless smile and vigorously scratches the indentations the mask has left on his cheeks.

"All you gotta do now is write them slips," he says. "I'll wait outside."

November 1989
July 1990
April 1991

"Yeah, I'm feeling good, just the cough and the itch, just like always. See?" Eddie coughs from the corner of the examining room, where he is checking out the soap dispenser over the sink. "You want me to sit down yet?"

"Just don't cough on my head." I have become used to Eddie's peripatetic habits in closed spaces like examining rooms, used to his incessant exuberant scratching and his loose-limbed speech, as elastic as a double-jointed thumb, but something about that juicy cough raining down on my head as I look through his chart still does me in. Fortunately, his good nature and desire to please seem bottomless. I could probably tell him to stop breathing while he was in my room and he'd do his best to oblige. So far I've settled for a ban on random coughing from a standing position without a tissue to catch the spray.

His chart is now filled with nine months' worth of my efforts to find him some more productive and treatable diagnoses than "chronic cough" and "chronic itch." I have been completely unsuccessful. All I've really done is satisfy myself within a hairsbreadth of certainty that, if he ever did have TB, he doesn't have it anymore and can't give it to others. The kids, now reclaimed back from foster care, are safe around that cough, and so, incidentally, am I.

He doesn't seem to have lice either, at least not anymore. The itch did actually get a little better after a trial course of an antilouse cream, but then it relapsed with a vengeance, and re-treating him didn't help. I've stopped every medicine he takes, one after the other, with no change in the itch. I finally sent him to the dermatology clinic last month, but they had little to offer. "Itchy bump syndrome," the clinic dermatologist has written in the chart, adding—possibly for lack of anything more helpful—"Severe!!" HIV-associated "itchy bumps" (prurigo nodularis to purists) are probably responsible for a greater quantity of discomfort than any other single feature of the disease. No creams or lotions stop the itch very well; no pills work at all. Some cases respond to hefty doses of ultraviolet radiation. Unfortunately, our hospital dermatologists have not yet invested in the equipment and personnel they would need to radiate all our itchy patients. Instead, sympathetically but firmly, they send them back to us to scratch.

The evaluation of Eddie's cough is stymied by a similar hospital quirk. What he probably has is a severe asthmatic bronchitis, exacerbated by the weather, the temperature, the humidity, the vacuuming of an old rug (and then, cruelly enough, the acquisition of a new one). Ordinarily I would send him for pulmonary function tests, which would give me some confirmation of whether this is in fact the correct diagnosis, and what medications might be helpful in treating it. But the hospital pulmonary specialists decided long ago that HIV-infected patients couldn't be tested in their pulmonary function machinery, which might trap infectious particles and transmit them to others. It's hard to argue with this kind of caution (although in other hospitals no such rules exist, and no infectious outbreaks have been reported from their pulmonary function labs). Still, the policy leaves Eddie the victim of therapeutic efforts on my part that are rather more random than absolutely necessary in this day and age.

So far, I can safely say that nothing has made him worse (except those rugs) and nothing has made him better (except disposing of them). He has cheerfully hacked through all of my ideas. Occasionally I become suspicious and decide that the problem must be that he isn't taking the drug of the moment, but his blood levels for the drugs I can check him for are always within the so-called therapeutic range. Therapeutic for everyone but him, that is.

"Telling you, always like this," he tends to say eight or ten times per visit. "Don't worry about it." Sometimes "it" refers to the itch, sometimes to the cough. "Status quo," my notes say now, a useful assessment that sounds more dignified than his but means about the same.

Status quo. He has a fraction of a fraction of a normal immune system, five T-helper cells at last count. Can this balancing act really be called the status quo?

But if I am unnerved by Eddie, he himself couldn't be happier. He feels good and he's putting on weight, so much weight that the teeth he ordered six months ago didn't fit and had to be returned. So the grin he flashes is still a yawning cavern, and his food is still puréed. But, as he points out, he orders out Chinese from his own phone and chops up the big pieces in his own blender in his own kitchen; his own wife wipes the counter and his own kids (actually, two of hers, two of his, and one of theirs) take out the garbage. For the first time in his adult life Eddie has got himself entirely in order. No impossible obligations are hanging over his head—no job that he's too high to attend to, no apartment whose landlord he has to avoid. Thanks in part to the city's beneficence toward people with AIDS, and in greater part to his own manic energy, he's straight, he's legal, he's rent-subsidized, and he feels good.

"Joined the day program," he says now, bouncing into the chair next to my desk. "Kids at school. Can't stay in the house all day. Like, a counselor or something."

The hospital's day-care program for AIDS patients, like similar programs for the elderly, aims to flush the housebound out of the house, gathering them for lunch, air, and activities. Eddie is hardly housebound, but neither is he, practically speaking, likely to find anything else to do with his time and energy. The cough and the itch would put off even the most generous employer. His wife, Lydia, is, as far as I understand, mandated by the child welfare tenets to be home full time for the kids. I glimpsed her earlier this afternoon, a plump redhead, surrounded by bulging shopping bags, waiting by the clinic copying machine.

"Lydia too?"

"Yep." He bounces up. "She made drapes for the room. We gotta go hang them now. You gotta refill the cough syrup. It don't do nothing but I gotta take something, right?" Big laugh. "I'm outside if you need me."

He vanishes briefly, then bounces back in. "Oh, yeah, I forgot, I gotta tell you, gotta tell you this, so we were all sitting around eating lunch, the first day at the program, OK? And so this girl over in the corner starts to choke, OK, and so she falls out of the chair and starts to shake all over and everybody is screaming so I says, I say, call the cops!"

"Great."

"Then I give her mouth to mouth."

"What?"

"Yeah, like I didn't really know how to do it but I hadda do something until the cops came, right? So that's what I decideda do. Didn't use no mask or nothing."

"Wow."

"So then the cops came and they take her over here, I guess. They said I did OK. So do you know, how'd she do, she do OK?"

In fact, I did hear some discussion in a meeting last week about Evelyn Rivera's seizure at the day-care program and her broken rib after six minutes of vigorous mouth-to-mouth resuscitation and chest massage at the hands of a hitherto unknown Good Samaritan.

"This is how I did it, just like this."

He is on the floor, pumping the tiles for a few seconds, then back in the chair. "Kids make me keep showing them over and over, won't let me quit. Pretty good, yeah?"

"Yeah!" There is no real need for him to know about that rib.

November 1989
July 1990
April 1991

October 1991

I know that cough. Sure enough, Eddie is at the door of the examining room, bouncing on the balls of his feet, fishing in one of his front pockets for a tattered piece of

Kleenex. I hadn't noticed his name on today's schedule. On the other hand, the schedule often bears little resemblance to the actual crowd assembled for medical attention at any given clinic session. Our patients are divided into two distinct populations, the ones who show up without an appointment because they feel sick and the ones who stay home and miss their appointment because they feel sick. We strongly encourage the former behavior and vehemently decry the latter, clear evidence that none of us working in the clinic is ever very sick. Sick—as I relearn for myself during my rare episodes of flu and food poisoning—is sick: sick is too sick to dress, too sick for the subway, too sick for the ambulette, and too sick to sit up for hours in anyone's plastic waiting-room chairs. Sick belongs in bed. If anyone belongs on the subway, it is Well, heading for Sick's bedside. But this is sedition. If you feel sick, come in to the clinic.

"Are you feeling sick?"

"Nah." He coughs again.

"Are you sure?"

"Yeah. Just saying hi."

"Oh, great. Hi."

He doesn't move.

"What's up?"

"Oh, yeah, well, you know not too much, just hangin' around. You know, I got like this itch behind my ear I just noticed, man, it's a bitch, you know?"

I know. He's had that itch since the day we met, the itchy ear that screamed "lice" so loudly I could barely remember my manners.

"I know. I know your ear. You've had that for a while."

"Yeah, I guess, a while."

I sneak a look at my desk, where Michael Soto's lab results are demanding some immediate attention and hard thought if he is going to stay out of the hospital for another week.

"So I thought maybe you could look at my ear, you know, just a look, like, I can't see back there. Or I guess maybe I could in a mirror. You got a mirror?"

He doesn't wait for assent but lopes into the room and over to the sink, where he perches on an edge and cranes to see behind his left ear. The red patch behind it looks exactly as per usual.

"Hey, you're going to break that sink right off the wall. Come on, get off. I'll look at your ear."

He ambles happily away from the sink and leaps up onto the table. I look behind the ear.

"Looks about the same. Are you putting the cream on it?"

"Nah. I gotta start putting the cream on it."

Another problem solved. "Do you need another prescription?"

"Nah, I got plenty." He shows no sign of climbing off the table. "Maybe you wanna listen to my chest too, you know, I'm coughing, coughing, coughing, it don't stop."

"You know, I'm kind of busy here . . ."

"Oh, yeah, yeah, I just been coughing, you know, coughing something terrible." He coughs his usual cough. "Maybe I should take an X ray."

"You want an X ray?"

"I took so many X rays, I'm gonna start glowing. My kids, they can use me for a night-light." He laughs a little hollowly. This is one of his favorite jokes.

"OK, so you don't want an X ray."

"Nah." He stays on the examining table, scratching behind his ear. He coughs. "You wanna listen to my lungs?"

I hear another chart rattle into my box on the door. I look at my watch. "You know, if you're feeling sick I'll definitely listen to your lungs. Are you feeling sick?"

"Nah, I feel good."

Then what, what are you doing here? I don't have time for you if you feel well. My time is diced up into tiny twenty-minute pieces and fed to the sick. None for you, unless you're sick—then I'll slice up someone else's piece and give half to you. Our clerk goes home at 5. The last ambulette leaves at 5:30. The clock is ticking. Two more hours. Six more patients. Up and down past my door nurses are patrolling, looking at the pile of charts in the door rack, looking at their watches. In the waiting room Michael Soto shifts on that rock-hard plastic seat, wishing for his bed. His sputum culture results are on my desk, and I have to deal with them now, this afternoon, ten minutes ago.

"You know, I don't have a lot of time this afternoon. Is the day care open?"

"Yeah. But I hadda be here. OK, so I'm gonna go, but I'm in the waiting room if you wanna listen to me, you know, to my lungs and all. I'm gonna go say hi to Mary."

"Good idea!" A very good idea. Mary's time is diced into even smaller particles than my own. Let her part with some of hers.

"See you. I see you in two weeks, OK? Two weeks. But I'll be outside if you need me."

"You bet. Two weeks. OK. Just close that door behind you."

But no sooner does the door click shut than it opens again. I wheel fiercely around, but it's only Mike Cook, one of the doctors enrolled in a special training program designed to give general practitioners hands-on experience in taking care of HIV-infected patients.

"I saw a new patient, her first visit to the clinic," Mike says. "Can I talk about her with you?"

Of course he can. The clock ticks on. Mike tells me about his new patient, very, very slowly. ". . . weight loss . . . diarrhea . . . no medical attention . . ." I try to speed him up just a tad. "No medical attention why?" "Oh, she has a lot of kids at home. And her husband, she says, is always sick, so she didn't even think about herself until the daycare program sent her over. So anyway, on physical exam . . ." Slowly, very slowly, Mike gets to the end. His patient is sick and complicated. Half a dozen young children in the house. Husband with questionable tuberculosis. Blood tests all out of kilter. Needs everything done at once. We rig together a plan for her. The clock ticks on.

But, of course, it's only when I head out to the waiting room, finally, finally, to liberate Mr. Soto from his bench, and I see Eddie sitting quietly, not a bounce, not a cough, not a scratch, whispering to a horrifyingly shrunken Lydia, that I slow down enough to catch on.

November 1989
July 1990
April 1991
October 1991

March 1992

I wouldn't have predicted that Eddie would so swiftly become adept at Lydia's wheelchair, maneuvering her in and out of the clinic with professional finesse despite the children sharing her seat, sometimes her blanket, leaping out to help drive, leaping back in to be driven. Not to mention the baby's stroller. The whole conglomerate arrives at the front desk like a battery-powered toy—the kind that never runs down—rattling, full of arms, drums, and noise.

"OK, yeah, here she is, here we are, give in the card, hey Nikki, give over your mami's card whaddya mean you ain't got the card? Look it looks like we mighta forgot the card but you know us right, I mean how could you forget, right. Ha! Hey there it is now give it in GIVE IT IN I SAID GIVE IN MAMI'S CARD there. So now we gonna sit right over there so if you need us that's where we are, OK?"

Then for the remainder of the afternoon the traffic to and from their waiting room encampment never stops.

The kids zoom up and away, on missions licit ("Quick! Mami feels nauseous, get a Pepsi from the machine quick!") and not ("Who tol' you you could bring that skateboard to the clinic?"), eventually settling in a corner with a couple of Mary's marking pens and forcible instructions to SIT and DRAW. Mike Cook fetches Lydia in the chair and delivers her back. Eddie comes to my door half a dozen times to say hi, to comment on the course of the afternoon, to pick up an extra prescription, to snag a quick opinion on a patch of itchy skin.

Today he has an appointment of his own. Lydia is in with Dr. Cook and Eddie is here with me, sitting shirtless on the examining table. Roughly a tenth of his attention is focused on what I have been telling him about his lungs. The rest has veered off to the racket outside, where a sudden clatter, a wail, and a tumult of raised voices have been only slightly damped by my closed door. Rubber-soled nurses' footsteps run down the corridor toward the waiting room. It sounds like the youngest Rios may have tipped over in her stroller again. The racket quickly subsides. Someone has picked her up. Rubber footsteps walk slowly back past the door.

"Crummy cheap thing always does that, hang anything, diaper bag, anything on the side, over it goes bang like that. Tol' Nikki and tol' her to hang that bag on the wheelchair not the stroller. I better go out take it off myself."

He shakes his head and prepares to jump off the table. If the fracas were still going on I wouldn't bother to stop him: by now the other patients are undoubtedly used to the sight of half-naked Eddie rushing out of my room to restore temporary order to his troops. But the nurses still don't like people without shirts in their waiting room, and they have been making increasingly sniffy noises about how they used to be working in a clinic and now find themselves keepers in a zoo.

"It sounds like things have settled down. Just stay here for a second, OK?"

Head cocked, he takes a reading. All is quiet. Nikki, almost eight, her stepfather's deputy in matters of household organization and discipline, has clearly managed to hang the bag elsewhere. Eddie struggles back up on the table and reaches for his shirt.

"What I gotta ask you is, she ain't eating, she don't even eat my spaghetti no more, and that used to be her favorite . . ."

"Wait, don't put your shirt on for a second. Stop talking and breathe."

Inhale. Exhale. Inhale. Then deafening noise—he's talking again. I have to take the stethoscope out of my ears.

". . . tried to give her ice cream last night first she says she wants it then she take a tiny bite and don't want it no more, so I tell Nikki to run . . ."

"Shhh. Just breathe for one second here." I put the stethoscope back in my ears, the diaphragm back on his chest. Inhale. Deafening noise. This is hopeless. I take the stethoscope out of my ears.

". . . four pounds last week so I call Cook yesterday, like I says, and I say, this is too fast. I know she's gonna lose weight but this is too fast. I say we gotta put the brakes on here, he says I'm right. He says it's the infection eating up her weight, eating up her food, he says that what happens, it's like I'm feeding her infection, it's like it eats up everything I cook. So she don't get none of it. That's what he says. So I say, we gotta put some brakes on here some way, you know? So he says I'm right."

He pauses for breath. I could probably whip the stethoscope back to his chest and get in a few more seconds of a lung exam, but in fact it's not really necessary. Eddie has become another one of my chronic bronchitics, always coughing, always wheezing. Ominous squeaks of pulmonary distress come through the stethoscope when he breathes. He's on and off antibiotics, with a small warehouse of "just in case the phlegm turns green" alternatives stockpiled at home. I decide to give up the pretense that listening to his lungs is a maneuver of any major importance. Better to hang the stethoscope around my neck and listen to him.

". . . so he says maybe she gotta go back in and strengthen up, but she says she ain't never going back in, so I says, baby, we gotta put some brakes on here . . ."

He knows as well as I do that there are no brakes for Lydia, whose vertiginous fall from health has dazed us all. Nine months ago she was sewing curtains and copying fliers for the day-care program. Now she is sitting in a wheelchair, barely moving as the five-year-old on her lap combs her hair. The histoplasma fungus roaring through her internal organs has been unstoppable. A trial of Amphotericin treatment in the hospital made her dangerously anemic. With transfusions and a lot more Amphotericin she might have had a chance, but Lydia is a Jehovah's Witness, no transfusions allowed. Now she is home taking pills instead, an alternate treatment that doesn't seem to be helping.

". . . she ain't going in, she ain't taking blood, so Cook says just make sure when she drinks the pills she drinks them with Coca-Cola so I say she don' like Coca-Cola, she likes Pepsi-Cola. So he says Pepsi-Cola's OK. So what I gotta know from you is, is the Pepsi-Cola OK, or I should pour the Coca-Cola into the Pepsi can for her to drink with the pills?"

"Pepsi's OK." Any carbonated beverage will give Lydia enough acidity in the stomach to absorb her medicine.

"OK, so I hadda make sure of that, I know you and Cook work together very close but just hadda check you know, and now I forgot just wait a second . . ." Out of his pocket he drags a grimy square of paper on which he has made a list.

"OK, so the Pepsi we got, and the hospital bed I did that already and the Ensure Mary gave me the case and Nikki's school I gotta do tomorrow and the dentist hey my teeth are ready been ready for a long time but I been busy you know, hope they don't give'em away. Ha! Maybe I'll go over there tomorrow no I gotta go with Nikki tomorrow she just wanna stay with her Mami but they say she gotta go back to the school. So I gotta do that tomorrow. OK so that's it, yeah, that's it."

"Wait a second." When he turned his list over to check the other side I recognized a familiar handwriting. "Wait a second. Isn't that one of your prescriptions?"

He pulls the wad of paper out of his pocket again and smooths it out. Sure enough, a prescription for Megace in my very own handwriting, written a month ago in the hope that this appetite stimulant might put a little flesh on Eddie's own bones. He is down to 125 pounds of nervous energy, thinner than the day we met. We have tried to get him as much household help as Medicaid will allow, but the major impediment to our good intentions turns out to be not Medicaid but Eddie. No stranger's cooking will do for Lydia: it's his spaghetti, his breakfasts, his touch in the tub she needs. He's sent back every aide and homemaker we've gotten him.

"Yeah, well, you know . . ." His voice trails off. He firmly wads his list back up and puts it back in his pocket.

"You told me you were taking those pills! And you didn't even fill it?"

"Yeah, well, I guess I thought I was drinking them but I guess I wasn't. I mean anyway four times a day pills, I can't drink those. I got no time to eat, how do I got time to drink four times a day pills to eat?"

He has a point.

"But listen. You have to take care of yourself. You know what I mean. You're not going to be able to keep this up. You could get sick too, you know? You have to start taking it easy. You know?"

Another crash and wail in the waiting room

"Yeah, well, I'll be outside, gotta go get that bag offa that stroller, I'll see you, OK, I'll see you later. Don't worry, I'll be OK I'm always like this, remember, status quo, remember, status quo, you taught me that, status quo right? Right?"

"Right. Status quo."

September 1992

November 1992

Anita Lewis

January 1993

SEPTEMBER 1992

The woman and the toddler who follow me into the clinic up elevator are both tiny and perfectly beautiful, out of place in that fluorescent cage of stubble and infirmity. Squeezed in the back, a sodden paper bag dripping my afternoon's coffee slowly through my fist, I idly watch the two of them. "Gimme some sugar," the mother croons, hefting the toddler up and nuzzling her up and down her neck, from ruffled pink sunsuit to tiny gold ear posts. She huffs a little from the baby's weight, one hand cradling the pink bottom, the other steering a pink stroller away from the glut of wheelchairs and walkers that crowds the exit. "Ooh, you're so heavy. Give me a old big kiss." A pleasant pastoral interlude before the storm.

Am I really surprised to find them in my examining room twenty minutes later? I suppose not.

"I was going to St. Hilda's," explains Mrs. Lewis, jiggling the baby on her lap. "It's a couple of blocks from where we live. I was in there for PCP last year. But I started to get the distinct feeling they didn't know what they were doing, so my husband and I decided I should come to a bigger medical center. So I'm here!"

Her enunciation is as exact as a television anchor's, her small chocolate brown face with its precise, chiseled, Anglo-Saxon features a perfect cameo in reverse. Her hair has been straightened and recurled into a carefully carefree tousle around her face; her makeup is tasteful and immaculate. She could be Miss America as she sits here, idly rebraiding the baby's back braid; she could be black Barbie, an ad for a household product, the lead in a situation comedy.

She has brought with her a neat package of medical records from the community hospital in Queens she has decided to forsake. It's hard to tell from the records whether they knew what they were doing with her there or not: she barely breezed by any of their facilities. Most of her clinic sheets are stamped Appointment Not Kept. She was in the hospital with a severe case of PCP last spring, signing out midway through her treatment, as soon as she could walk without an oxygen mask. Her last T-helper-cell count, measured almost a year ago, was 15. In the six months since her pneumonia she made a few clinic appointments at St. Hilda's and kept none of them. She dropped by a few months ago for a medication refill. That was it. It's not the attendance record you would expect from such a perfect profile, such exact locution and precise dress.

"So, you didn't get to your other clinic too regularly, I see?"

"Oh, I have been so bad about that! I really do feel badly about missing all those appointments. I'm going to try very hard to do better here, believe me."

"What medicines have you been taking?"

"Well, frankly, I've been awfully bad about that too. I ran out of everything . . . let's see, it must have been a month or two ago. And I was really too embarrassed to go back and get more."

"Embarrassed?"

"Well, you know, I had decided to come here, and had asked for my records and all. So I felt I really couldn't ask them for anything else, it wouldn't be right."

All this is delivered with the most gracious and charming of smiles, self-deprecating shrugs inserted in all the right places. At one point, a kiss on the baby's head. Clearly, what we have here is the muse of Miss Manners'

Guide to the Life Threatening Diseases: be polite in your quest for important medications; try not to be a burden to your institution of record.

"So you haven't taken any Bactrim in, say, three months? Would that be right?" Bactrim is the drug that treats PCP and keeps it from recurring. Unlike many of the treatments used for AIDS, Bactrim is (at the moment, at least) fairly uncontroversial: it's cheap and it works. Even the vitaminists, the macrobioticists, and the other devotees of nontraditional therapies grant Bactrim a grudging respect ("I take my vitamin A, my vitamin C, my vitamin E, my zinc, my selenium, my blue-green algae, my ginseng, and my Bactrim"). About 50 percent of HIV-infected people are allergic to Bactrim and have to take some less effective medication like pentamidine or dapsone. But for the ones who can tolerate it, Bactrim is a lifeline. Without it, the majority of people who have had one episode of PCP will get it again within a year or two. With it, the risk of recurrent pneumonia is greatly reduced.

"Yes, let me see, I suppose three months is about right. It took a long time for this appointment to come through. It didn't seem right for me to just show up and ask you all for prescriptions."

Of course not. After all, we hadn't been introduced. A brief vision flashes through my mind of the scene at the clinic counter on some Friday afternoons, the bellowing hordes shouting "You gotta give me . . . ," "I gotta get . . . ," until the clerk loses patience and slams off for a break. Not a scene for Miss Manners.

"And how have you been feeling?"

"Well, now, there's the thing. I'm glad you asked that question."

Were we going to talk about our hobbies?

She fishes a toy for the baby out of her tote bag and concentrates on her answer.

"Until last month I felt great. But recently I haven't been feeling entirely well. That is the truth, and I've got to admit it. The problem is with my breathing. I cough from time to time and I'm having a hard time catching my breath sometimes. Coming here I had to stop twice on the landings of the subway stairs with the stroller. It was terrible, so many people backed up behind me! But I just couldn't go any further. And then I was fine. After I rested. For a while. And fever. Too."

What she says is worrisome, but the way she says it is a flashing red light of emergency. This woman is clearly becoming short of breath just talking an uninterrupted paragraph. I can't spend the rest of our time together asking the routine questions about her path to HIV infection and her medical history. This is an emergency, and I don't even have to think very hard to figure out what the problem is most likely to be. She stopped taking her Bactrim months ago, and her PCP is on its way back.

"You catch your breath for a minute, and I'm just going to listen to your lungs." Sure enough, as in most cases of PCP her breathing sounds normal through the stethoscope, with none of the squeaks or silences that might suggest other problems. Her chest X ray will probably be entirely normal. But I've seen enough PCP to smell it a mile away.

"So I would bet this is the way you felt before you went into the hospital with PCP."

She thinks for a moment, then nods. "At the beginning, now that you mention it, I guess it was. It got a lot worse, of course, before I went in. My husband doesn't like my being away from home. He just. Goes crazy. So I tried. To hold out. But I couldn't." She stops abruptly, takes a few breaths of air.

Well, now, isn't this going to be fun. She has got to go right back into the hospital. No one who gets that short of breath describing how short of breath she is should be farther from an oxygen canister than a yard or so of plastic tubing. If I knew her better I would be able to negotiate with a little more finesse; as a well-meaning stranger I'm sure I don't have a prayer. In ten seconds we're going to be locked in the ring in mortal disagreement.

"You know, I can tell from looking at you just how short of breath you must be getting."

"It's not really that bad. It's just very close in here, you know, stuffy." Ah, nice return. This is going to be lawn tennis rather than women's wrestling.

"Still. I have a sneaking suspicion that your PCP is on its way back. What do you think?"

A gracious, rueful smile. "You know, I think you might be right."

"You know, Mrs. Lewis, when someone gets this short of breath from PCP, it's usually a good idea for them to be in the hospital for a little while, just to get some oxygen and make sure that the treatment takes effect the right way. You know what I mean?" What I mean is that you may well gasp to death at home unless you get some treatment right now, is what I mean.

The smile is even more gracious, but the shake of the head is regal and unmistakable.

"Oh, I knew you would say that. But I just couldn't. I'm terribly sorry. It's out of the question."

Game and match. We look at each other. For an instant a blind raises in her eyes and I see a whole range of reasons why she doesn't want to be away from home.

"Why is it out of the question?"

The blind snaps down. She laughs, rolls her eyes. "Oh, he is sooo helpless! Can't do a thing for himself! You know men."

I sure do. But I'm not going to know hers, not if she has anything to do with it.

I make her sign the hospital's Refusal of Recommended Treatment form to absolve me and the clinic of any legal responsibility should something go awry. These forms sometimes frighten patients into reconsidering their decision to go home. Not her. I'm not surprised. I put together a package of second-best alternatives for her: blood slips, a chest X-ray form, a prescription for Bactrim pills. I deliver the usual warning: "People get a lot of stomach upset from taking the number of pills I want you to take every day. If you can't get them down, or start to feel worse, you should come back here right away. Or go to the hospital near you. Either way, I want to see you next week. OK?"

"Oooh." She makes a little face. "It's such a long way! But I will definitely try to make it! Definitely! And thank you so very much for all your trouble! Say thank you to the doctor!"

The little girl stares at me blankly. I stare back.

September 1992
....

November 1992
....

At first I actually thought she might come back when she was supposed to. Then, after a few phone calls that rang unanswered at the number she had given us, I thought she must have been admitted to the hospital in her neighborhood. Then, after we sent her a telegram to call us and no one replied, I knew she must be dead. Then she came back.

She's thinner than she was six weeks ago, but even more perfect, groomed and curled, stockinged and heeled. And all alone.

"I'm so glad to see you!" And I am: a weight in the back of my mind that no Refusal of Treatment form ever really takes away has just dissolved. "Where's the baby?"

"Thank you! It's so good to be here again! The baby's with her grandmother. I just put her over there for a little while, you know, so I could do some good cleaning. Without her underfoot. You know babies!"

She is smiling, animated, and breathing very quickly.

"We were worried about you. Did you ever get our telegram?"

"Why, yes, of course. I was so touched by that, I can't tell you. It was a lovely thing to do! And I'm so very sorry I didn't have a chance to get back to you, I'm so bad about things like that. But I was thinking of you, don't you worry. And now, here I am!"

Yes, here she is, fluttering as hard as ever she was trained to do. (What military academy of manners did this to her? How could anyone interpret our stock "Call the clinic immediately" telegram as a lovely gesture?) And here, unfortunately, am I as well, earthbound and faced with the ugly job of netting this ethereal sprite, pinning her to my board, and figuring out what in the world she is up to.

"So I guess you're feeling better?"

"Oh, ever so much better!"

"How did you do with the Bactrim?"

"Oh, I couldn't take that dose of Bactrim! I tried as hard as I could, but I'm afraid it was just impossible! My stomach just wouldn't obey."

I knew it.

"Ah. Remember I told you to come right back if that happened?"

"Oh, it's such a long way. And I didn't want to bother you with my little stomach problem. So I worked it all out myself."

"You worked it all out?" This is going to be bad.

"Yes, what I did is I took two or three pills every day. Instead of six. That way they lasted much longer. In fact, I just finished them. So that's why I came back; I had promised myself. I was going to try to be better. About my medications."

"Ah."

A long dead silence ensues. She pats her hair and catches her breath. I look at her chart. I feel very tired. I don't know what to do now. It would be pointless to mention that if two or three Bactrim pills a day treated PCP, I would have told her to take two or three pills a day. All that dose of antibiotic does is dampen the disease a little, mute it, distort it, the same thing that happens with any other infection you treat halfway. It may look like it's going away, but it's just gone around to jimmy the kitchen window while you're still locking up the front door.

"Are you still coughing?"

"You know, it's good you brought that up. I was going to mention that. The cough has become terrible. At night I can't stop. My husband makes me go over to the sofa so's he can get some peace!"

"Are you having fever?"

"Well, I must admit, I was going up to 104, 105 a few weeks ago, so what I did is, I stocked up on Tylenol and cough syrup at the Rite-Aid. I probably had a touch of the flu. The fever doesn't go nearly so high anymore. And the cough is a little better too. I'm afraid I've run out of both of those, though, if I could trouble you. I understand they come in prescription form."

I'm starting to think that she must actually be crazy. Despite the elegant grammar and manners she must be insane. There is no husband, no grandmother, no house to clean. She has come straight from a lunatic asylum to torment me. She borrowed the baby as a prop and left it in a stairwell when she was done with it. She isn't a patient at all. She's a plant, a ruse. Perhaps I'm back in medical school and she the actress playing my problem patient for Clinical Interviewing and Diagnosis. The intervening years have all been a dream.

"It looks like you've lost a little weight." She has lost fifteen pounds in the space of six weeks.

She smiles again, but whatever she plans to say is lost in a spasm of coughing. "Start to cough when I eat," she mumbles finally from behind a wad of Kleenex she has taken from her purse. "Needed to lose a few pounds anyway."

I can't stand any more of this. I send her downstairs for a chest X ray.

When she comes back, freshly lipsticked and smiling, passing me the slip from the radiologist that announces that her X ray is negative, I know she's preparing for a fight. How I would love to just call it a day right here, patting her on the coiffed little head and sending her home with a sincere "Be well!" or "Feel better soon!" or "Take care of *you!*" Unfortunately, I am paid to be the straight man here. The kindly and euphemistic approach didn't work last time. This time I'll be more direct.

"Listen to me. Even though the X ray is negative, the PCP is still there. That's why you're feeling so bad. Or

it may not be PCP. It may be something else just as serious. Either way, you have to come into the hospital and
get treated properly. There's no other choice."

She smiles, but for the first time she's stopped flirt-
ing. Under the lipstick she is cast iron. "I told you, I just
can't."

"You know, this is a life-threatening infection we're
dealing with here. It's not a cold. It's not the flu. You can
keep it suppressed for a while, but not forever. You have
to get treated the right way. Will you go into the hospital
near you? Shall I call them?"

"I told you, I just can't. But it's very nice of you to be
so concerned."

"Can't you tell me what's the problem? Maybe we
can help you with it, get a sitter, a homemaker . . . ?"

I can tell I'm not on the right track here. It's not
dustballs that are the problem. Now she's sneaking a look
at her watch. She has to be going. Back to clean house?
Back to pick up the baby? Back to bed, most likely, to rest
up for another day of . . . what? I can't even imagine the
possibilities. She has plunged in and out of our clinic so
abruptly and dramatically that none of the usual intake
interviews with the nurses or the social workers has taken
place. I don't have a clue how she came by her HIV infection. If the baby is HIV-infected. If the husband is. All I
know is that she is gathering her things together. It's getting late. Thank you for a lovely time.

"Oh, and I need some kind of a cream for a discharge too, if you would. In my, you know, down below."

"A discharge in your vagina?"

"Yes, just, you know, whatever cream you would use for a little sore."

"Well, that kind of depends on what you've got down there. Let's have a look." A sore and a discharge could mean a dozen things, from candida to syphilis to herpes.

"Oh, no, I just don't have time for that. Just give me whatever cream would do the best job."

"Mrs. Lewis, I can't do that. No cream will do a good job for everything. I won't do a full exam, if you don't want, but I've got to take a look."

"I'd really rather not."

"It's your choice, then, but I can't give you anything to help." This is not disciplinary action on my part: I would actually be happy enough to oblige, but I would honestly not know what to give her.

She sighs, gets up on the table, pulls down her underclothing, closes her eyes.

"Oh, my God." The words are out before I can stop them. Her vaginal area is a mass of sores, oozing and crusted. She has the worst case of vaginal herpes I have ever seen. I can't imagine how she is able to talk, let along walk, without any sign of discomfort.

"How long have you had that for?"

"Just a while." Her eyes are still closed.

"Did you ever have that before?"

"A few times."

"This bad?"

She nods.

"Did you take anything for it?"

She shakes her head, adjusts her clothing, climbs down from the table, avoiding my eyes. "You can give me something for it now? I really do have to be going."

I look at the pad of Refusal of Treatment forms for a while, and then decide to forget it. I write her out prescriptions for clindamycin and Primaquine pills, different drugs for PCP that are easier on the stomach than Bactrim and almost as effective. They actually usually lead to diarrhea rather than nausea, but maybe she'll make it through a couple of weeks. I explain to her how to take them. I write her out a prescription for acyclovir capsules for her herpes. I tell her to come back in a week. She nods and smiles and thanks me copiously for everything. I am quite sure I will never see her again.

"Mrs. Lewis?"

She turns back from the door.

"I have to fill out some forms on every new patient. Would you mind telling me how you think you got your HIV?"

She smiles gently. "I don't talk about it. But thank you for asking. It's good to know. That someone cares."

September 1992
November 1992
....
January 1993
....

They tell me that a passing nurse took one look at her and led her right out of the line at the registration desk, half-walking her, half-carrying her down to the treatment room at the end of the hall. By the time an aide gets me out of my room to come see her ("Doctor, Mrs. Lewis's early for her appointment, but they said to tell you she don't look so good"), she is sitting on the edge of one of the recliners where our patients get blood transfusions and intravenous medications, leaning forward, shoulders hunched up, gasping. One of the nurses is reading the instructions for hooking up the oxygen canister. Another is covering her with a blanket. Mrs. Lewis looks up at me.

"Here. I. Am!"

Here she is, two months after she was supposed to come back, a vision in PCP. She's clearly in no state to answer many questions, but that doesn't matter, because I don't really have anything much to ask her. Maybe she took some of the pills I gave her, or maybe she didn't take any of them. Maybe she breezed by her neighborhood hospital, maybe she didn't. Maybe she even went somewhere else, to a new neighborhood, a new hospital, where maybe she told them the real problem and maybe she didn't, where maybe she was, just for an afternoon, any ordinary pretty young woman with the flu, looking for some Tylenol, some cough syrup, some reassurance. Whatever maze she's been wandering in the last few months, it doesn't really change where she's ended up, oxygen mask now green and jarring against that perfect face.

A person who comes down with PCP for the first time has, with the proper treatment, about an 85 percent chance of getting well. The more times they have had PCP, the worse they do with each episode. The harder they are breathing when their treatment begins, the worse they do. The more medicines they've tried without success for an episode, the worse they do. Mrs. Lewis has maybe a two in three chance of leaving the hospital alive, maybe one in two, maybe one in three. Whatever it is, it's substantially less than it was the day we met.

A woman leaning against the back wall of the treatment room holding a tangle of coats, bags, and scarves approaches me. "You gonna keep her, right?" I look over at Mrs. Lewis, expecting some weak volley of protest, but there is nothing. She just looks back at me.

"I'm her sister. We tried to get her here sooner but she said she had an appointment that was for today and she didn't think it was right for her to be showing up out of turn." The sister is heavy and cheerful; she looks nothing like the drooping butterfly on the edge of the chair.

Mrs. Lewis nods confirmation. "Called for. Appointment. Last month. This was. Earliest."

Have you ever heard of an emergency room? Or even an ordinary telephone? Has your sister? I just nod.

The sister goes on. "This is some flu, right, Doctor? Is this that Hong Kong we been hearing about?"

Mrs. Lewis's eyes are widening in panic. With all the strength she can muster she is vigorously shaking her head, eyes fixed on mine. For a moment I'm confused. Then I recognize that panicky signal. I am not to say what she has aloud. Her sister doesn't know, doesn't know a thing. Her sister thinks the infectious disease clinic exists to take care of the flu. And I'm not to tell her, I'm to let her blithely stumble on.

"She had that bad flu last year, when she was in the hospital. She say that might have been the Hong Kong. But this one's gone on for much longer. This is normal, to be getting this flu every year? Maybe she needs a shot. I got the flu shot at work this fall. But Anita, she don't work, so she don't get it automatic-like. Maybe that's the problem."

She leans back against the wall, satisfied. Mrs. Lewis's eyes are still fixed on mine.

"We're going to keep her and make sure she gets treated for what she has," I say carefully. I haven't been in this kind of a situation for a long time. AIDS is far less often the closely kept secret from families that it used to be. When someone is left in the dark now it's usually a sexual partner. In those cases we sometimes step in and break the news ourselves, justified by the ethicists and the law in sharing the secret to protect the uninfected at risk. But if the unenlightened family member is not at personal risk—a parent or an in-law, often—we try not to breach our patients' confidentiality, even if it would be to every-one's advantage to do so. Usually siblings prove to be valuable allies and confidants for our patients. But Mrs. Lewis, of course, is not what you would call the confiding type.

"I'm gonna go make a call, then," says the sister. "I'll call Mom to keep the baby till I get there, then I'll take her back to your place, like we said."

Mrs. Lewis smiles faintly and watches her out of the room. Her breathing has slowed, and she is now leaning back in the recliner. The machine the nurses have hooked up to one of her fingers to measure the quantity of oxygen in her blood is flashing and beeping: her value is 91 percent and has set off the machine's danger alarm. She's going to need to go to the intensive care unit with a value like that. One of the nurses switches off the alarm signal, but the display keeps flashing silently.

"You're going to stay with us this time?" I reach over and hold the oxygen mask away from her face so I can hear her answer.

"I guess. I have. No choice."

"Who'll take care of the baby?"

"My sister. Will stay over. Take care of. Them both." The voice is suddenly breathless and bitter. But when the sister comes back into the room, two coats and two hand-bags draped over one arm, a soda from the vending machine by the telephone in the other hand, the smile behind the mask is back in place.

Shannon Gallagher

JULY 1989

The clinic is going through one of its periodic summer staffing crises, and Susan Pollock has arrived to help. At least, this is the intent of the decision that has moved her one afternoon a week from the hospital's methadone clinic over to us. Susan is a nurse-practitioner who usually spends her time refereeing the stream of medical complaints offered by the methadone patients as they pick up their daily dose. She has leapt at the opportunity to escape from behind the methadone counter for a few hours each week, and we are happy to get another functioning practitioner for busy Wednesdays, even though her contribution will probably be, at least for a while, more theoretical than actual. She is inexperienced with many of the more serious illnesses we see, and by law she has to discuss all her cases with a supervising physician, which means she will be occupying a fair amount of someone's time today.

That someone appears to be me; it's the middle of July, high vacation season, and I'm the only doctor in sight. But Susan is an enthusiastic trainee, happily picking up charts and calling patients back into her cubicle, emerging a reasonable amount of time later to discuss the case and have me sign the chart. Most of her patients have been uncomplicated, and the afternoon has progressed without incident.

And now I'm wondering what's happened to her. It's been over an hour since I last saw her, heading out to the waiting room with a fat chart under her arm to call someone's name. In the meantime I have finished seeing the last of my own patients, the waiting room has cleared, the sun has lowered on the horizon, the nurses are covering up the supplies and locking the doors—and Susan is still closeted with someone in her examining room. Who does she have in there? I want to go home. The reception desk is empty. I tap at Susan's door.

No answer. I tap harder. The door cracks open and Susan's face, looking oddly swollen and teary, appears.

"You OK in there?"

"Oh, yes," she says thickly, clearing her throat. "We just got to talking. I'll be out in a second."

"Who do you have in there?"

"Shannon Gallagher. I'll be right out." The door clicks shut.

Of course. Shannon the pathetic, the eloquent, the articulate, recently discharged from a six-week hospital admission. No wonder it has taken so long. An appointment with Shannon can take up an entire afternoon. Between her hair-raising medical problems and her compelling personality, she personifies the pathos and tragedy of the young, victimized, and dying better than anyone I have ever known. By rights she should be lobbying Congress, but instead she has had to settle for a smaller circle of admiration within our walls.

I first met Shannon about eight months ago, during one of my assigned months working at the public hospital down the street. At the hospital's "AIDS attending" that month, I spent my weekday mornings on patrol up and down the hospital's inpatient wards, checking on the AIDS patients to make sure they were receiving up-to-date care and answering any HIV-related questions the hospital's nurses and doctors might have. In the middle of one quiet morning I got a page from the psychiatrist on duty on the hospital's locked ward, where actively suicidal or threatening patients were confined until they calmed down. A patient, admitted a few days ago after a suicide attempt, had just told them she had AIDS. Could I come up and give them some advice on what to do with her?

Early that afternoon I was buzzed into the locked ward and shown to Shannon's room. Nothing was visible but a mound of blankets on the bed. When I knocked at the doorframe, a tiny, woebegone face emerged from the heap, and a sudden sweet smile broke through. "You must be the AIDS doctor," she said, turning over and sitting up. "Thank you so much for coming to see me." I was instantly charmed.

Shannon told her story clearly, precisely, and chronologically. All I had to do was listen. It was a familiar one: she had grown up in a well-to-do family in the suburbs, discovered drugs in her early teens, left home, moved to the city, worked as a prostitute to support herself, got her high school equivalency, took some college courses. ("I liked psychology," she said, "but what I really wanted to be was a veterinarian.") Fell in with a bad crowd, began to live with an addicted, abusive boyfriend. Tested HIV-positive five years ago, but was too drugged out to get any consistent medical care. Developed PCP, diagnosed with a lung biopsy at Pelham Hospital fourteen months ago. Was treated with Bactrim until she developed a violent reaction to it ten days into treatment and was switched to pentamidine. After she left the hospital she had become more and more depressed, and after a beating by her boyfriend last week had become actively suicidal and came to the hospital for help.

"I told the other patients at the group meeting last night that I had AIDS," she said in a voice barely more than a whisper. "Maybe it was my imagination, but I thought they all began to avoid me afterward. So I asked to be moved to a private room. I feel safer here. I know I have a bad disease. But I'm still a human being!"

Just turned thirty-one, Shannon was tiny, skeletal, and didn't have a tooth in her head. Her hair was thinning, her face pockmarked, and her arms and legs scarred from years of heavy drug use. The rest of her physical exam was encouragingly normal. She had the enlarged lymph nodes in her neck, armpits, and groin that result from both intravenous drug use and HIV infection; otherwise, everything seemed to be in order. All I had to suggest to the psychiatrists was that she begin to receive some basic HIV medicines while she was in the hospital, and that she be referred to a good HIV clinic when she was discharged. I had our own clinic in mind. Shannon was a compelling and enjoyable person to talk to, and she knew her medical history so well that the endless and irritating process of obtaining medical records from another hospital wouldn't be necessary with her.

I talked to the psychiatrists and went back in to let Shannon know what I had recommended. She happily agreed to inhale some pentamidine to prevent recurrent PCP, but she was a little dubious about AZT. "They told me at Pelham I wasn't a candidate for it because I had a bunch of kidney operations when I was a teenager," she said. "And anyway, I decided a while ago that I'm not really interested in anything that will prolong my life without really adding to its quality, you know?" I knew. I agreed we would hold on the AZT. I gave Shannon our clinic's phone number so that she could make her own appointment if the psychiatrists couldn't get through.

Four months later she showed up, triumphant. In the time since her discharge, she said, she had landed in another Bronx hospital with a second episode of PCP and a pelvic infection. Then she had lost the phone number I gave her. But she had asked around on the streets, had got the number, had made the appointment, and had appeared. She was pleased as punch with herself and ready to turn over a new leaf. No more street drugs, she promised, no more episodic, discontinuous medical care. She needed someone she could trust to do something about her headaches.

The headaches were disabling, increasingly frequent and severe, and none of the usual tests showed anything abnormal. After a few weeks she began to complain of some numbness in her right arm and leg, and a few weeks later she had definite weakness on the right side of her body. We put her in the hospital for a careful neurologic assessment.

And now here she is, two months later, in Susan Pollock's examining room with a thick new hospital chart. When the door opens and Shannon heads out into the waiting room, I can see she is still limping. I had lost track of her in the hospital, although occasionally I heard from some of the nurses what a rewarding patient she was to take care of. ("So sensitive. The things she says, they'll break your heart.") From her limp, it seems like the six weeks hadn't been much of a success.

When Susan and I, sitting side by side, finally plow through the important parts of her chart, it is clear that, far from being a success, Shannon's hospitalization was a travesty, one disaster after another. All her scans and spinal fluid tests were negative during the first week of her admission. The neurologists couldn't figure out what process was causing her right-sided weakness and numbness, and without identifying the problem they couldn't recommend a solution. But even so, everyone wanted to do something to help Shannon. So Shannon's kindly intern began prescribing potent narcotics for her headaches. Shannon's kindly dietitian endorsed her request for hyperalimentation, the high-calorie intravenous feedings one of her roommates at Pelham had received. A kindly surgeon promptly put a plastic intravenous catheter into one of the big veins in Shannon's chest.

In fact, when these catheters are used for high-calorie feeding they almost always get infected, which is why we rarely use them unless we really have to. For a person who can eat and digest, swallowing calories is much healthier than having them infused. Sure enough, after a few days of intravenous feeding, Shannon suddenly developed a high fever. She had an abscess where the catheter entered her chest and all kinds of bacteria growing out of her blood: a rip-roaring catheter infection. She was given antibiotics for a few weeks. The catheter was pulled out and another one was put in. She was scheduled for discharge, then just the day before she was supposed to go home, she was again found barely conscious with a temperature of 106°. Another abscess was oozing on her chest wall, and more bacteria grew out of cultures of her blood. The catheter was pulled out and not replaced. She was given more antibiotics. Then everyone realized too late that she had become addicted to the high-dose narcotic pain relievers she was getting for the headaches. She wound up having to enroll in the hospital's methadone program to get off the pills.

"Wow." Susan is shaking her head as we get to the last page of the record. "I've been seeing her at the window over at the program, but I never talked to her before. She literally had me in tears in there. Did you know that when she left the hospital the floor nurses actually gave her a party? She's really proud of that. She used to help them make beds, on her good days. She wants to die with dignity, she says, to make up for wasting her life. She has terribly low self-esteem. I'm sure her boyfriend is still kicking her around. She has a little yellow-green under one eye that looks like it used to be a shiner, but she won't admit it. I guess he's all that she's got, really. Here, can you sign my note?"

Susan's note is excellent and complete. She has refilled Shannon's vitamins, her pentamidine, and the AZT Shannon has begun to take in the hopes it might alleviate her headaches. She has filled out slips for Shannon to have some follow-up blood cultures done, to make sure the catheter infection is completely cleared, and some other routine labs.

"No T cells?" Since Shannon already has a diagnosis of AIDS, knowing the number of T-helper cells in her blood won't change the medications we prescribe for her. This is why we often stop doing expensive T-helper-cell counts once a patient gets a disease, like PCP, that gives them a diagnosis of AIDS. Still, we find that many of out patients insist on knowing their "T-cell number" anyway.

"No T cells," Susan says, gathering the papers together and looking at her watch. "She doesn't want them. She says that since she already has AIDS they're meaningless, and anyway they're usually so low they just depress her."

Just the kind of intelligent prudence I would expect from Shannon. I head out to the waiting room to say hi and welcome her back to the clinic.

July 1989

October 1989

"I'm sorry I didn't go. It just seems so pointless. I sit down there for an hour sometimes before they call me, then they have to poke around for a vein . . . I hate it. You remember what I said when we first met—I just want comfort-type care, not aggressive-type? I guess that's why I don't feel more strongly about getting them done . . ." Her voice trails off in a sigh.

Shannon has been more than a little remiss about getting her blood tests done. She loses the slips, she has urgent appointments that don't permit the wait, and now she has skipped straight to the theoretical underpinnings of laboratory tests and is meditatively trying to explain to me how blood electrolytes conflict with her philosophy of end-of-life care.

I am about as sympathetic as I can ever be to people who fool around with their blood tests, but I still don't buy it. The capsules and pills we lavish on our patients are almost all miniature time bombs. One patient in ten or a hundred will develop reactions to them that may become life-threatening or permanently disabling if not picked up in time. The complications of HIV, another time bomb, can sometimes be anticipated and minimized by timely blood tests too. Blood is a vital part of the unwritten contract binding us all together in our strange, troubled marriage of the ill and the well. Without blood, everything begins to fall apart.

Still, it is difficult to speak sternly to Shannon as I would to any other patient, and banish her to the laboratory to get her blood drawn before she gets any appointments, any attention, or any medications—our version of finishing spinach before getting dessert. Dealing with her is, eerily, just too much like dealing with a professional colleague for this sort of discipline. She continues to impress us with her precise knowledge of HIV, of the medications she takes and their potential side effects. Frowning in concentration, her plug-ugly little face a sunken apple-doll without its teeth, her scanty hair permed into droopy ringlets, she follows her own course with the clinical detachment and interest of a professional.

"I see my Babinski's still there," she is apt to remark as I scratch the bottom of her right foot with a key and watch her toes fan up and out in abnormal response. "Dr. Marley didn't check it last week, but when Dr. Hill checked me last summer before I was admitted it was there." Her abnormal Babinski reflex is just one of her alarming neurologic unexplainables, along with the incapacitating headaches and the right-sided weakness that have persisted and worsened since her hospital discharge. In fact, her Babinski reflex (a "pathological reflex" in the language of the neurologists) is one of the few clues in her puzzling case, and it's not much of a clue at that. All it indicates is that somewhere on one of the major nerve highways between brain and right foot something is amiss. The scans and the antigen and antibody tests that usually can pinpoint where the problem is and what's causing it have all been completely unhelpful in her case.

Still, Shannon has done remarkably well in the months that she's been out of the hospital. Her weight has increased by ten pounds, she is on a stable dose of methadone at the program, and she insists that she is through with street drugs. Her spirits usually seem good, although the black depressions that landed her on most of the locked psychiatric wards in the Bronx still surface from time to time. In fact, she was back in the psychiatry unit of Pelham Hospital across town only a couple of months ago. But that was a short stay, terminated at her own request. When she was released she proudly brought me a copy of the letter she had written to the physician in charge of her case there, and asked that a copy be filed in her record with us too, "just in case":

"I am requesting my discharge as soon as possible," she had written. "As a voluntary patient I am permitted the right to request my discharge. True, I have been depressed, but not unduly so. I wouldn't do anything to harm myself. Nature is taking care of that. I belong home. What is left of my life should be spent trying to be happy and comfortable. The thought of spending any more time in hospitals (than is medically necessary) is intolerable. I do not believe that staying in this environment is healthful to me mentally, emotionally, or physically. Please inform me of your intentions as soon as possible. Respectfully submitted, Shannon Gallagher."

Since then, Shannon has chattered to the nurses and the other patients at great length about her moral triumph at Pelham Psych. She has not mentioned the fact that two days after her discharge she was back in our emergency room with a shattered jaw, courtesy of the boyfriend who is part and parcel of the home where she belongs. She had called the police and moved some of her possessions out of the house but apparently just couldn't bring herself to press charges. Now she sports the odd bruise every so often, but only once has she linked bruise and boyfriend. "He gets angry when I don't take my AZT," she admitted a few weeks ago when one of the nurses asked her directly what was going on. "He really loves me." She had no interest in receiving any kind of protection from his love, and the subject was dropped.

It's hard to square her evident intelligence with this kind of psychologic blindness, but she is hardly a unique case of this particular inconsistency, and so it is even more difficult to play the bad guy with her. Today she's a little yellow under one eye again and looking particularly woebegone.

"Look, Shannon, you haven't had any blood tests since you left the hospital, that's more than three months ago." And she didn't have so many in there either; between the constantly infected catheters, the state of her veins, and the sympathetic intern, she had got away with the bare minimum.

She looks sad.

"I know they have a problem with your veins sometimes, but go down and try. I'll have your prescriptions ready when you get back."

"I better get the prescriptions now. I've got an appointment in an hour—I'm going to start volunteering at that soup kitchen for HIV patients at St. John's."

"I'll have them ready when you get back."

She looks at me hard, really hard, for a second, an unexpected flash of hostility from one of my pet patients. Then I remember the bruises (and, once, what we think must have been cigarette burns) dotting her arms when she hasn't taken her AZT in the past. My carrot-and-string games with her medications may actually be life-and-death maneuvers for her.

I almost tell her to forget about the blood tests, but the words stick in my mouth. Then the moment is over; she picks up her slips and limps out of the office.

"I'll give them two tries," she says, "and that's it. After that I'm leaving."

That seems fair enough to me.

July 1989
October 1989

January 1990

"I gotta get the straight story here. I'm fucking sick of being jerked around here!"

A massive tattooed forearm suddenly begins to slam down onto my desk—but it stops, trembling, every muscle rippling, within a millimeter of the surface and lowers itself silently down. That's the last straw for me. My examining room door is already open as wide as it can get, but before I even think about it I find myself up out of my chair and standing in the doorway. If I'm going to be murdered, it might as well be within full sight of a witness or two.

The big, angry person attached to the fist now lying on my desk has accompanied Shannon to the clinic this afternoon and has asked to speak to me. This is hardly an unusual request. It's the rare patient who doesn't, sooner or later, show up with a friend or family member who wants to draw us aside for a hurried private conference. These conversations are never a lot of fun, ranging as they do from "Now let me ask you right out, he doesn't have (pause) *AIDS,* does he?" to "I called the funeral home next street over and they said they won't do her; is that allowed?"

It very much looks as if this session is going to be one of the worst. Shannon is in the waiting room reading a patient education brochure about cholesterol. She only shook her head when I called her name and beckoned to her a few minutes ago, and in turn beckoned me over to where she was sitting next to this enormous leather-jacketed stranger.

"My friend Jack wants to talk to you," she said. Would she like to come in and be part of our conversation? "She knows what I'm gonna be saying to you, she don't need to be there," answered friend Jack, rising to his full height and preceding me down the corridor to my room.

Should I escape out to the hall phone and call Security? One more slam of that fist and he's gone, as far as I'm concerned. Meanwhile, I'll just stay over here by the open door. Unfortunately, my fight-or-flight posture isn't likely to do much to calm him down. One of the cardinal rules of talking to patients about bad news or threatening subjects is to sit down, or at least, the experts say, make sure your head is lower than theirs. This posture apparently does more than all the words in the language to reassure of good intentions. When pressed, we are all lions and jackals and sheep.

"What, uh, do you mean, uh, by that?" I am perched half in and half out of the room, the doorknob digging a hole in my back. I should be sounding firm, unruffled yet sympathetic. Instead, I sound like a sheep.

Jack, fortunately, isn't listening. His eyes are closed and he is very evidently trying to control himself.

"Look. Do she got it or not?"

"It? Uh, AIDS? Uh, yes, I'm afraid . . ."

He cuts me off. "Yeah, OK, I know. I know she got it. OK. So why don't she get no treatment?"

"No treatment? But she does get treat—"

"She don't get nothing regular. And she don't take nothing regular. So what I want to know is, who's dicking who around here?"

"Look, uh, Mr., er, Jack, you'll have to watch your lang—"

"Sorry. I apologize, Miss. But I just don't get why she don't get no steady supply of medicines."

Hmmm. Steady supply. An attention-catching way of putting it, I must say, with definite mercantile overtones. Might some of Shannon's AZT be winding up in Jack's pocket for a little street-corner dispensing? Not, actually, that she's had much AZT recently. The blood problem came to a crisis three months ago when the phlebotomist in the lab downstairs missed twice, could milk only one tube of blood out of the third try, and Shannon returned to the clinic in tears. "I just can't go through any more," she whimpered. "Just give me my prescriptions. Please?" We gave her two weeks' worth of prescriptions, but she's been giving us a wide berth since. She must have run out of her supply months ago.

"She never took the TZ regular, and now she don't take it at all. And when I ask her, she say you all quit giving it to her. But what I think is, I think it's her playing around again. I told her, this was Christmas week, OK, I told her to get right back here and get her medicine. And if she's not supposed to be taking the TZ, then find out why not. And the breathing treatments likewise.

"So she says, OK, she'll find out and she goes to get on the train—but I follow her to the train, see, behind her, and I watch and there she is coming up on the wrong platform, and there she is getting right on into the wrong train. So she goes downtown, she thinks I'm dumb or something.

"So when she gets home, I say, did they explain about your medicine? So she says, they don't want me to take it no more. So I say, why not. So she says, because I'm dying that's why. So I say, look, I know dying. Dying takes more medicines. Not less. So I tell her I know she's lying.

"So I say, I'm gonna go there with you, I'm gonna take you there, and this Dr. Zulu she's gonna explain right to me, right to my face, OK? So like I says, you all better level with me, Miss."

In the middle of this speech I have half-closed the door and slunk back around into my chair. Jack's eyes are open now and his head level is safely above mine, but I have lost all sense of alarm. This is just too much like a scene from *West Side Story* to be personally threatening. This character in black leather is no street-corner pharmacist, and he has no interest in damaging me whatsoever. The entirety of his interest, benevolent and otherwise, is clearly focused elsewhere.

"Shannon has made some decisions about what medicines she will and won't take—"

"Yeah, I heard that, that's all garbage. Gar-*bage*. She's sick, she gotta take medicines. I know she won't get no better, OK, but you're sick, you take medicines. That's the way it gotta be. So I just got her so she take that TZ, just like it says on the bottle, every four hours on the dot, no forgetting, no dropping it into the wastebasket or into her pocket, no nothing, and so now she ain't getting it no more?"

"No, we would very much like her to keep taking it. It's just that—"

"What the fu . . . I knew she was di . . . screwing me around, that . . ."

"Hey!" One of my forefingers has risen of its own volition, and I seem to be on the verge of shaking it in this maniac's face. Not a good idea at all. I put the forefinger down. "That is, I mean, why don't you just let me explain one thing?"

It doesn't take long to fill him in with an edited version of Shannon's blood-test problems. I leave out any implications that her skittishness is voluntary or irresponsible. I ascribe it all to the sorry state of her veins, although I am not myself entirely convinced that this is the case. I give a lot more credence to her quite sophisticated concepts of comfort-oriented end-of-life care, but I don't bring these up either. As far as Jack is concerned, he explains again, sick needs medicine, very sick needs hospitals, and dying needs more of all of them.

"Before she went, my mother got maybe thirty, forty kinds, and she took them all." I have every reason to suspect that Jack was instrumental in this ingestion. And I have a feeling that, were I to suggest Jack draw Shannon's blood himself, nothing would make him happier. Instead, we reach more of a theoretical understanding. He will simply encourage her to keep her appointments and cooperate with us, taking what is prescribed and submitting to what is ordered with as much precision as possible.

"OK, so I got it now." Jack is rising and pumps my hand. "I got everything straightened out. Nobody's going to do no more di . . . uh . . . scr . . . uh, no stuff no more. You can count on me, Miss. So you want I should send her in now for her blood?"

I hate to pass up this opportunity, but I'm more interested in Shannon's blood results when she's been taking her medications rather than when she hasn't.

"We'll do it next time."

Jack nods and disappears. I have a sudden thought, fleeting as a bad dream, that I have neglected in all the excitement to bring up the agenda we usually try to review whenever a sexual partner appears on the scene:

protection, precautions, misconceptions, and the partner's own state of health. For a moment I think about calling him back. Then my good intentions fail me. I did well enough with Jack today to feel satisfied, if not downright smug. Next time, I think. Next time. Or maybe not. Dr. Zulu may not actually be the ideal person to head unarmed into a discussion of Jack's personal life, lion tamer though she may otherwise be.

July 1989
October 1989
January 1990
April 1990

"Come with me for a second."

Shannon follows me obediently out of the little examining cubicle, out of the waiting room, and into the main corridor, a hundred-foot stretch of empty hallway. A few patients waiting on benches beside the doors to other clinics watch idly as she walks down the length of the corridor, turns, and comes back to me. There's no question about it. The limp is more pronounced, and her balance seems to be off as well. Her gait is broad-based, as if she were straddling a long puddle, to compensate. When I ask her to walk heel-to-toe along a straight crack in the linoleum she almost falls over. She has just told me she's noted more weakness in her right leg and arm, and the headaches are worse than ever. Last night, she says, she had a fever of almost 103°.

Back in the examining room she picks at the torn knee of her blue jeans.

"I almost forgot, I've got to tell everyone in the waiting room about the jeans place," she says suddenly.

"The jeans place?"

"This church in my neighborhood got a special donation of extra-small jeans for AIDS people. Sizes one and three. It's really hard to find those sizes in regular stores. See—Gitano size one. I'm going back today for more." She stands up and pirouettes, a little off center, and has to steady herself on the edge of the desk. The jeans are close-fitting and impossibly small, the waist perhaps the size of one of my thighs. I check her chart, and sure enough, her weight is down again, she's barely a hundred pounds.

"And I found a place where they give you free cheese if you're HIV too. I gotta tell everyone that too."

"Are you eating? Do you have an appetite?"

"Yeah, I eat. Sometimes." She pauses, still standing next to the desk.

"So that's it for today?"

This catches me by surprise. In my long experience with deteriorating patients, they seldom tell me cheerfully that all their symptoms are worsening, start running fevers, lose ten pounds in the course of a month, then make for the door. Usually it's just the opposite: the sicker they become, even if we all know that nothing more can be done, the more they want to stay, talk, and be examined. They need the ceremony of the encounter. Usually they actually have to be pried out of the examining room. But here Shannon is jiggling by the doorknob, all unconcern.

"Um, wait a second. Sit back down for a second."

"I really have to go, you know?" Now she is jiggling on the edge of the chair. What is up here? She's not depressed again as far as I can tell. She may well be back on drugs, if she ever got off them, but she's not high at the moment, neither irritable nor drowsy nor drunk. Certainly not demented. She just wants to go shopping.

"You know, it seems to me from examining you and watching you walk that the weakness and balance problem *are* getting worse. I'm worried about your fever. And this weight loss worries me too."

I seem to be alone in this emotion.

"So does that mean you'll give me a cane?"

"Well, yes, sure, I can write you for a cane, but I also think it may be time to do a few more tests to see if we can figure out what's going on here." It's been six months or more—I have actually lost track—since the last scan of Shannon's brain failed to show up any abnormality that might account for her symptoms. Last month, escorted downstairs by Jack, she had a set of blood tests that looked fine. But the phlebotomist managed only two tubes for the routine blood counts and chemistries, none of the more esoteric serologic tests that might help diagnose this progressive neurologic process.

"You want me back in the hospital?" Jiggle, jiggle.

"Well, now, how would you feel about that?" ("I belong home. What is left of my life should be spent trying to be happy and comfortable. The thought of spending any more time in hospitals is intolerable . . .")

She considers for possibly two seconds.

"Yeah, I guess, OK. But not today. The jeans were almost gone yesterday and I want another pair. I'll come in tomorrow, OK?"

This is getting stranger and stranger. I need a little time to think it all over, and to talk to the social worker who works closely with Miss Gitano here and might have some insight into this turn of events. I also need to put together a reasonable plan for repeating her neurological workup. Plopped into the hospital without a careful plan, she is bound to be plopped right out again by the overworked residents on the wards unless I give them a blueprint of action.

"Well, I'll tell you what. Why don't we repeat one of your scans as an outpatient first, just to get things started, and then talk about the hospital. OK?"

She actually shrugs. "Doesn't matter to me. I'll wait for the papers." She's out of my room in a flash.

It's hard to believe that hesitant, broad-based wobble got her into the waiting room so fast.

But this thought doesn't reach my conscious mind until later.

It surfaces at the end of the afternoon, to be precise, four hours and five patients later. All the patients have gone home and I am now blearily finishing their paperwork. The last thing to take care of is the requisition form for Shannon's MRI scan. I have to fill out a detailed questionnaire, and I'm also going to have to call a neuroradiologist tomorrow and get approval for the test. Since the neuroradiologists are apt to be curt, to put it kindly, if the facts of a case are not laid out to their liking, I pick up Shannon's three-volume chart and start reviewing it from the beginning. I realize with a start that there are whole sections I've never looked at at all. I never have any time, is the problem. I'm always rushing from one patient to the next, from a meeting to the clinic, from the clinic to a meeting. I can never spare even the half hour a close reading of this pile of paper is going to take. I might as well make the most of the experience and take some notes—Shannon is clearly going to start being an active patient and I'm going to need her history at my fingertips.

At the end of forty minutes I have a sheet of notes that read very differently from the way I thought they would.

I have the formal reports of two CT and two MRI scans of the brain, all entirely normal.

I have three complete sets of blood tests for the most common neurologic infections in AIDS, all negative.

I have a consulting neurologist's report that her "degree of subjective weakness cannot be confirmed on objective testing."

I have the brief note of one of my colleagues who saw her while I was on vacation last summer: "Her exam seems exaggerated. Her Babinski reflex seems almost voluntary."

I have set after set of remarkably normal blood counts. ("Good news, Shannon, your red and white blood cell counts are almost normal!")

I have a patient who never gets thrush, although she never takes medicine that might prevent it.

I have a patient who has never gotten another episode of PCP, although she rarely shows up for her pentamidine treatments to prevent it from recurring.

I have no medical records from the hospitals where she did have PCP.

I have no T-cell results. ("They just depress me.")

She twinkled out of my examining room so quickly this afternoon. Did she limp? I was too busy looking for a requisition form to notice.

Those infections in her catheter. Those lymph nodes. That Babinski. Those blue jeans. I don't know what to think.

July 1989
October 1989
January 1990
April 1990

June 1990

Shannon has an appointment today. For six weeks she has not been out of my mind. I have lived her and breathed her, as obsessed and disbelieving as a lover, as methodical and vengeful as the law. She has an appointment today. I know she won't be here; in fact, I don't think I'll ever see her again. But I'm still waiting for her. For the past week I've been looking over my shoulder, expecting to see her heading toward me with a weapon, with her bare fists. I'm afraid she's going to kill me. Or have Jack kill me. She has an appointment today. I couldn't sleep last night. What will I do if she shows up? What will I do if she doesn't?

It has been more than two months since I put down her chart after reading it cover to cover and, with a vague feeling of unease, filled out her requisition for another scan of her brain. It was a week later that, yet another normal scan under her belt, Shannon had limped back into clinic. She looked pale and distraught. Her balance was going fast, she said. She had a bruise on her forehead where she had fallen onto the sidewalk the day before. Her headaches were worse than ever. She had had to buy some Dilaudid on the street to numb them a little, she said. She was ready to come into the hospital.

We took another walk down the corridor outside the clinic. This time she couldn't go even ten feet before she began to teeter from side to side so violently that I had to run up and steady her. Back in the examining room she said she was too weak to hoist herself up onto the examining table and sank instead into the chair by the desk. Her right arm was pathetically weak, as was her right leg and the grip of her right fist. She could barely manage the laces on her sneakers when I asked her to take off her shoes and socks. Her reflexes checked out as usual: her knees and ankles bounced normally when I hit the tendons, but that classically abnormal Babinski reflex was still present in her right foot, the toes fanning out dramatically when I kneeled down to scratch the sole. I ran my knuckles down her shinbone—another, less frequently used way of checking the same reflex that I had looked up in an old textbook the night before. Her toes curled smoothly under: a normal response.

She watched. "What's that one for?" she asked. If an intelligent person is around doctors and hospitals enough, and asks enough good questions, she's bound to learn all about reflexes. I scratched the sole of her right foot again. Her toes performed their abnormal response perfectly—right out of a textbook. I ran my fist down her shin. Her toes reacted perfectly normally.

"What's that one for?" she asked again.

"Nothing special. I'm going to draw your blood myself today, Shannon," I said. "Maybe we'll be able to keep you out of the hospital after all."

"Thank you, I appreciate that." She closed her eyes. "I need time to finish my living will before I go back in."

I grabbed a fistful of tubes from the supply closet and a tiny flexible needle that, to my surprise, slid with no difficulty whatsoever through her scarred arms into the large veins underneath. I wondered briefly about those problems the technicians in the hospital lab were supposed to have with her veins. Then I sent Shannon off with her social worker to finish her living will.

When the contract of trust disappears, it goes like smoke. Left with the bouquet of blood tubes on the desk, I had no difficulty in allocating them for the tests I wanted. I sent a set for T-cell studies and specimens for all the other tests Shannon had been missing for so long. What plenty, what luxury. At the end, one red-stoppered tube was left over.

My debate with myself lasted a few minutes, but it was no contest from the start. By the letter of New York State law, I need signed consent from a patient before I can send blood for an HIV test. I am forbidden to order the test without it. But this policy is intended only to protect the HIV-infected from being identified without their knowledge or consent. The spirit of the law has no interest in protecting the rights of the HIV-uninfected who have, whether by accident or design, been mislabeled. I was still breaking the law. But I didn't really care. I filled out an HIV-test slip for the remaining tube of blood and delivered it to the lab myself, before I could change my mind.

The T-cell studies were the first to come back, three days later. Shannon had 1,250 T-helper cells per cubic millimeter of blood, entirely within the normal range. An AIDS patient with her history would be expected to have no more than 200, probably considerably less.

Her negative HIV test took three weeks to return.

First I thought that, possibly, long ago, some doctor had made a terrible mistake, had been misled by Shannon's scrawniness and her swollen drug user's lymph nodes, had told her that she must have AIDS. Then I remembered her confident, brave little voice reciting the details of all the AIDS-related infections she had had at other hospitals, all so precisely diagnosed that they could have been taken from a textbook. Her Babinski reflex, so abnormal it could have been taken from a textbook. Her textbook concepts of death and dying.

I went into high gear. I was possessed. I called the Department of Health labs where all the HIV testing in the city is performed and asked them to test her specimen again, and also to test it for variant types of HIV that the standard test may not always identify. I called her social worker, who confirmed that Shannon had indeed just completed her living will, and that Jack had given her another black eye last week. I called a friend of mine at Pelham Hospital, where Shannon had had her first episode of PCP. He pulled her chart from the record room. I took half a day off from work to trek across the Bronx and pick it up.

Shannon never had PCP at Pelham. Shannon never had any kind of pneumonia at Pelham. Shannon had never gone to Pelham with anything having to do with AIDS at all. She had been seen in their emergency room a dozen or more times over the past seven years, saying that she was passing a kidney stone and asking for the potent narcotic pain medicine used to treat that condition. She was seen in their psychiatry emergency room half a dozen times for depression. Last summer she had indeed been admitted to their inpatient psychiatry unit for depression. She told the psychiatrist there that she had been treated for PCP at my hospital several years before, by me!

I went to two other Bronx hospitals. Both had charts in her name. They contained no records of PCP, or pneumonia, or weakness, or headaches. Just depression, kidneystone pain, and demands for pain medication. Even during the last fourteen months of our acquaintance she had been shuttling in and out of other emergency rooms in between her clinic appointments.

I begged Dr. Ortega, one of the hospital psychiatrists who had met Shannon during her hospitalization, to come talk to the clinic staff at an emergency meeting. She was calm and philosophic about the whole thing. Everyone else in the room looked as if they had been struck by lightning. Shannon's social worker was clutching her copy of the living will.

"Factitious illness has many variants," Dr. Ortega said. "Some patients fabricate illness for pure secondary gain, narcotic pain medication, say, or social service entitlements." Or blue jeans, methadone, free cheese.

"In other cases the secondary gain isn't so obvious. Many of these patients were deprived of love during childhood. So they wind up looking for and finding the love and attention they crave in the health-care system. They subject themselves to medications, operations, infections, anything to stay in that nurturing health-care environment. But of course they can't stay too long, or they'll be discovered. So after a while they make themselves unpleasant, stage scenes, disrupt hospital routines, and vanish. Then they turn up somewhere a thousand miles away, and go through the same thing. These are the patients with classic Munchausen's syndrome.

"I must say, Shannon is pretty unusual, to have stayed around so long, to have gotten along with you all so well."

"We loved her!" blurted out one of the nurses.

"That's what I mean," Dr. Ortega said gently.

Shannon clearly couldn't keep coming to our clinic. For one thing, she needed far more psychiatric help than we could provide—although the psychiatrist predicted that she would never accept it. Patients with factitious illness are notorious for eluding psychiatric care as compulsively as they seek out other kinds. The problem with banishing her from the clinic immediately, though, was clear to those of us who had met Jack. He was likely to murder her if he found out what she had been up to. No one had any good suggestions for resolving the situation, but the first step was clearly to get Shannon's consent for another, aboveboard, HIV test, a basis for whatever was to come next. And it was clear whose job that was.

When Shannon limped in for her next appointment, an electric current traveled the clinic. No one looked at anyone else. Mary put the chart in my box without comment. I called Shannon in before all my other patients, although I usually operate on a strictly first-come, first-served basis. My hands were shaking.

"How are you doing?"

"About the same." She was matter-of-fact. "How did the tests come out?"

"Well, actually . . ." I took a deep breath. I had rehearsed this so many times it sounded almost natural.

"Well, actually, I have some good news for you! The tests came out very well. In fact, some of the tests of your immune system were very strong. Almost normal!"

I braced myself, but she didn't move. Instead, she smiled from ear to ear.

"You're kidding! That's wonderful! Maybe I'll beat this thing after—"

"In fact," I continued relentlessly, can't stop now, "in fact, they're so normal that I think perhaps we should repeat your HIV test. Just to see what version of the virus you have. It may be a very unusual one."

This was pure invention on my part. But she nodded soberly. We signed the forms, all clean and legal. She rolled up her sleeve. In a moment it was over.

"The results will be back in three weeks," I said. "I'll see you then."

She smiled over her shoulder as she left. After a few seconds I looked out to the front desk. She was there, making her next appointment, a bandanna fluttering gaily out of the back pocket of the size-one Gitanos. Then she wandered out of the clinic and down the main corridor to the elevators. I followed and watched her from our doorway. The limp was gone.

And now it's three weeks later. Her second HIV test is as negative as her first. The time for her appointment has come and gone, hours ago now. All my other patients have come and gone. The volumes of her fat chart are stacked on my desk. Finally, I turn off my light and leave too.

José Morales

SEPTEMBER 1991

"Where is Dr. Grossman? Has something happened to Dr. Grossman?"

Mr. Morales's face falls when I call his name in the waiting room, and as he obediently follows me back to my cubicle he loses no time in cutting to the chase. He has been coming to see my colleague Dr. Grossman since time immemorial (actually seven or eight years would be closer to the mark, but among our patients that length of days is a geologic age), and the rheumy eyes behind thick wire-framed spectacles are wide and worried.

"No, Mr. Morales, don't worry, he's fine, but he's gone on a sabbatical. He'll be away from the hospital for about six months. So I'll be looking after you until he comes back." And curse Dr. Grossman, last seen with a broad smile creasing his face as he packed up his desk and headed off for a semester at a research institute in London. He might at least have mentioned to his patients that he was staging a small disappearance from their lives and not leave that chore to others. But then, those on the luscious verge of jumping ship, however briefly, have been known to forget to look back.

"Oh." Mr. Morales is still standing, looking panicked, as if he's just lost his wallet.

"It's only for a few months, Mr. Morales."

"Oh."

"I'm sorry. It'll be OK, really. He'll be back before you know it."

"OK." He pauses, sits down in the chair, glances wildly toward the closed door.

"Remember last summer, when he was on vacation, and I filled in for him? That wasn't so bad, was it?" Indeed it wasn't; we got along just fine. I always kind of liked Mr. Morales, which is why I volunteered to adopt him for the duration of Dr. Grossman's British adventure. Why is he looking so dismal?

"It's just that, I been having some difficulties," he finally blurts out.

He shows no signs of going on.

"Well, perhaps I'll be able to help you with them."

Or perhaps not; perhaps I'll never hear what they are. Mr. Morales is now deep in silent misery, twisting his hands together and looking off into the distance. To my great disbelief, tears seem to be welling up into his eyes. Really, is this called for? It is not. The next six months just got a lot longer for the both of us. Perhaps I will take this opportunity to leaf through his chart for a few minutes and leave him time to regroup.

Only about three years' worth of Mr. Morales's history is in the thick folder I have in front of me. The more remote parts are contained in coded files long buried in dusty filing cabinets in the research wing of the hospital. He is a patriarch and a pioneer among HIV patients, a long-term survivor not only of the infection but also of the hospital's ground-breaking epidemiologic studies, begun almost a decade ago, of HIV-infected drug users and their heterosexual partners. These detailed tracings of sexual connections across the Bronx were among the first studies to demonstrate to a disbelieving scientific community that HIV could be spread by heterosexual contact.

I remember listening several years ago to some of the research nurses reminiscing about how they got to know Mr. Morales. It was a sometime girlfriend of his, diagnosed to have AIDS, who enrolled in their study and listed him as one of her casual sexual partners. He was contacted several times by the nurses and finally agreed to participate in their interviews and blood tests. He later referred his wife into the study, and another girlfriend also surfaced. Were there other girlfriends? I can't remember. But I do remember the final mapping of his particular circuit of HIV clearly: Mr. Morales and both girlfriends were infected; his wife was not.

The actual path the virus took among them was, of course, untraceable. Mr. Morales, a casual drug user at the time, may have acquired his infection from a dirty needle and passed it along to the statistically predicted 50 percent of his sexual partners. Or the girlfriend may have been infected by another association and infected him in turn. Or a long forgotten former girlfriend of Mr. Morales's may have spread her infection to him and some of his other partners. Or Mr. Morales may be, despite interview after interview, nonjudgmental question after nonjudgmental question, a man who has had sex with men but has removed himself so far from this behavior as to actually have put it away from his memory, an experience not forgotten so much as disowned. Gay pride is notoriously absent from many segments of the Hispanic community.

"Who did this to me? I bet I know who it was." For all the research into the transmission of HIV, these knotty tinders of pointing fingers, flying accusations, burnt-out lusts, forgotten memories, remain as impenetrable as ever. One mention of HIV and they ignite into flash fires scorching through whole landscapes of family ties and friendships. However it was with them all, now almost a decade ago, today's reality will not change: Mr. Morales's girlfriends are long gone, his wife is home with their two young children, and he is sitting here in my chair, small, plump, middle-aged, excesses of his past all, I'm sure, a fading memory, misery etching new lines on his face as he contemplates the desertion of Dr. Grossman.

Looking over the past few months' worth of notes, I am developing a theory about why Dr. Grossman is being so desperately mourned. It may have a great deal to do with Dr. Grossman's innate understanding of the prostate gland, which seems to be the source of all Mr. Morales's current problems. Of HIV-related complaints, he has had literally none, although his T-helper cells have been waning for years. On the other hand, his blood pressure is up, he is getting a little arthritic, and his prostate has been behaving like the prostate of any fifty-five-year-old man.

"Still up to urinate 4–5 times per night," wrote Dr. Grossman last month in his delicate angular handwriting. "Hesitancy and dribbling." He has ordered the necessary urine studies, treated Mr. Morales for a possible infection of the bladder and the prostate, and arranged for him to get an appointment with the urologists. Has Mr. Morales gone to see them? Only Mr. Morales knows.

"So, listen, Mr. Morales, it looks like everything's been OK except for the urine. Did you get to the urologists yet?"

The eyes, still misty for Dr. Grossman, now fix on mine.

"The urine doctors? Did you see them?"

"No, I don't . . . I don't think so."

I look at the back of the blue plastic card clipped to the chart where a list of his appointments is kept. His urology clinic appointment was ten days ago.

"It looks like you missed the appointment with them."

"Oh."

"Mr. Morales, are you still having problems with the urine like you were telling Dr. Grossman last time?"

"You know about that?" His eyes widen. He reaches up and nervously adjusts the little leather cap he always wears.

"It's in your chart. Mr. Morales, are you feeling all right?" He has never been the most animated of men, has always seemed far more geriatric than his years, a ruminant figure in a guayabera shirt sitting in a corner of the waiting room much as, I imagine, he sits on a folding chair in front of his apartment building in the summer, watching things go by. But he has never before been this vague and bizarre. He's coming to pieces in front of my eyes. Or maybe it's all the modesty of a middle-aged man's first confrontation with his prostate.

"I feel all right. Except for the, you know, the . . . you know."

"The urine?"

"Yes. The urine."

"Well, so that's why Dr. Grossman wanted you to go to the urine doctors."

"I see."

"Was there any reason that you didn't go?"

"Well, I . . . I wanted to stay with Dr. Grossman."

Ah.

"You know, he wasn't sending you there forever, Mr. Morales. Just for them to look at your prostate. You know, a visit. A consultation. Dr. Grossman wasn't getting rid of you."

"Oh."

"You understand what I mean here? Mr. Morales? Are you with me?"

"I should go to the urine doctors."

"Yes. And you should come here too. For the HIV."

"Ah. I got the HIV too?"

Oh, my. Much as I might like to, I can't blame this lapse on Dr. Grossman's forgetfulness, or on Mr. Morales's modesty. Last summer he knew exactly what he had, not to mention who I was and what I could be expected to know. No one could endure the battery of tests and questions accompanying enrollment into one of the early HIV epidemiologic studies and not know all about his own HIV infection, not to mention those of occasional others.

"I'm afraid you do, Mr. Morales. Remember that study up in the other part of the hospital, with Kate and the other nurses?"

"Yes."

"Well, that was all about the HIV. Remember?"

Evidently not. "I see," he says, considering. "So that's how it is."

"Look, Mr. Morales, I'm going to ask you a couple of questions, OK?"

"Yes."

He knows the date, the president, and the name of the hospital. I am Miss Zuger, a lapse so standard I have decided that I can no longer in good conscience count it as a wrong answer. He has no headache, no fever, no weakness or numbness of arms or legs, no drooping of the face.

He could be depressed. He could have a quiet infection in his brain. He could have any number of things, but I'm pretty sure I recognize the signs of HIV eating holes in brain cells, leaving only empty space behind.

"Are you sad about anything, Mr. Morales? Is anything bothering you?"

"No, not really." And in fact, he doesn't look sad. Just blank, depleted.

"Did you come to the clinic alone today?"

"No, with my wife."

"Can you go get her and bring her in for a second?"

"She's downstairs in the car. Double-parked."

"Can she come up for a second? I want to talk to her for a second."

"She has to stay with the kids and the car."

"I really have to talk to her for a second. Can you go down and stay with them and send her up?"

"OK, I'll go down and tell her. I should tell her you want to see her. Is that right?"

"That's right. Just for a second." Just to ask her what's happening at home, to warn her what may happen, to make sure he keeps the appointments for the tests I'm going to schedule. "Then I'll send her down and you come back up."

"I see."

He leaves and I wait, but I have made a foolish and major tactical error. She never comes up. He never comes back.

September 1991

March 1992

"Hello, Mr. Morales."

"Hello, Doctor."

At some point during the last six months I graduated from Miss to Doctor. I don't think that it was all those blood tests or scans of the brain that did it; I was still Miss long after we established that no process other than HIV was chewing through Mr. Morales's memory. It certainly wasn't his ill-fated morning in the urology clinic, where, unaccompanied and far too shy to discuss his problem with strangers, he spent a bewildered morning, bewildered everyone who talked to him, and made a quick escape. I may have turned into Doctor on the afternoon when, following some broad hints dropped by Mr. Morales, I deduced that he was becoming impotent from his blood-pressure medicine and substituted another one. His air of quiet panic and perplexity seemed to subside after this intervention, and he stopped counting off the months till Dr. Grossman's return, at least in my presence.

"How are you feeling?"

"I feel OK."

"What's new?"

He obediently searches his mind for items of newness. Nothing seems to fit the bill.

"How's the urine?"

He nods. No effort on my part will get him back to the urologists, not even offers of going with him to their clinic and making sure they understand his not very difficult to understand problem. One morning of strange women asking personal questions was enough. There have been no more urine complaints out of him since.

"Nothing doing?"

He shakes his head politely. I begin my standard review for people who, like rusty pumps, have to be primed to complain.

"Any headache?"

No headache.

Blurry vision?

No blurry vision.

Trouble swallowing?

No trouble swallowing.

We proceed slowly downward, through breathing, chest pain, stomach pain, diarrhea, and winding up, again, with the urine. He considers carefully. No, no problems with the urine. He reminds me of an obsolete personal computer I have at home, so slow that you can actually watch it think, grind painfully through calculations that the newer ones do without a break in the pattern of the screen. I harbor persistent suspicions about Mr. Morales's prostate and urine, but without the cooperation of the prostate's owner all my kind concern is immaterial.

"So everything's all right."

"Yes," agrees Mr. Morales after some thought. "I think so."

"Hop up on the table and let me take a look at you."

He clambers up onto the examining table without too much effort and perches there uncertainly, still wearing his leather overcoat and leather cap.

"Why don't you take off your coat? And take off that hat too for a second, while you're at it." Dr. Grossman is scheduled back next week, and I want to return Mr. Morales to him in a polished and presentable state. For all I know he is hiding a case of something awful under that hat he never takes off, and if so, Dr. Grossman will never let me forget it.

"I should take off my hat too?"

"Just for a minute."

Very reluctantly, he removes the shiny leather cap. There is nothing more insidious underneath than a small, balding skull, feathered over with the soft hair of the HIV-infected. I know no explanation for why HIV does what it does to body hair, thinning and wisping the locks on the head, sometimes lengthening the eyelashes to incredible degrees. Patients turn into incarnations of urchins painted on velvet, heartbreak guaranteed. Mr. Morales's eyelashes are not yet at heartbreak length, but the downy bumps of his skull are almost equally devastating. I can understand why he never takes his cap off and have to hold myself back from recommending that he never do so again. The rest of his physical exam progresses with the hat firmly in place.

"So. Everything seems fine."

"Yes, Doctor." He edges himself off the table.

"How are things at home?" I've never had even a glimpse of Mrs. Morales, who is always downstairs in a double-parked car, but she has talked to Mary on the telephone several times, and my understanding is that she is managing to cope with his increasing hesitancy and forgetfulness without too much anguish. It is unlikely at this point that he will ever recover his lost mental ground. Occasional reports, when AZT was first released, told of dramatic reversals of HIV dementia on the new drug, but Mr. Morales has now been through AZT and DDI both with no improvement in his condition. If his disease follows the usual course he will just keep slowing, like a sticky cassette tape or a miswired computer, until eventually he slows to a halt, apathetic, mute, and bedbound.

"How are things at home?" Mr. Morales, distressed and far away, isn't answering. Is he suffering from another potency problem?

"Mr. Morales?" His eyes are misting behind the thick glasses.

"I been having some difficulties. But she'll be back soon."

"Who'll be back?"

"My wife, she went away somewhere. She took the kids. But she'll be back soon."

"Where did she go, Mr. Morales?"

"She didn't say."

This could be as trivial as a visit to her sister or as catastrophic as a body buried in the backyard. There's no way of knowing from his blank despair.

"Are you managing OK by yourself?"

"I been busy fixing up the house so it'll be nice when she gets back."

"Are you eating?"

"I can't cook. I go out to McDonald's to eat."

His weight seems to be holding up. "Well, don't tire yourself out now, OK?"

"Yes, Doctor. Thank you, Doctor."

He shrugs on his leather coat and trundles a little uncertainly out of the office. I make a beeline for the nurses' station, where Mary is taking a temperature.

"Have you talked to Mrs. Morales recently?"

She moves me out of earshot of the thermometered patient. "She called while you were in with him."

"So?"

Mary can deliver devastating news utterly deadpan; I think she may have taken a course in the technique.

"She said she thought we should know she's in a safe house."

"A safe house?"

Mary moves to take the thermometer out of the patient's mouth. "Go have a seat in the waiting room now." She moves back to me. "She says Mr. Morales poured boiling water on the little boy."

"Oh, no. What happened?"

"That's all she said."

"Can we call her?"

"Nope." Safe houses, to protect women and children from vengeful mates, have strictly guarded telephone numbers.

Mary takes another chart from the rack and turns toward the waiting room, where a dozen patients wait to be interviewed, weighed, and have their temperatures taken.

"Wait. Wait. This is terrible. What do we do now?"

"She said she's not pressing charges. She just wanted to get the kids away from him."

"Oh, God." How glad I am that Dr. Grossman will be taking over this situation.

"I told Paul he had to talk to him today." Good idea. Our social worker Paul is a reliable storehouse of practical advice. And in fact, as Mary and I move out into the waiting room, I glimpse Mr. Morales trailing after Paul into his cubicle down the hall.

Forty minutes later Paul is at my door with a handful of forms. "ASAP," he announces, plopping them in front of my nose. They are for visiting nurse service, home care service, and a homemaker to visit the Morales home. I fill them out on the spot.

"What happened, did he tell you?"

"He says they had a misunderstanding." Paul rolls his eyes, recaptures the forms, and disappears.

I follow him back out to the waiting room where Mr. Morales is gathering up his things to leave.

"Mr. Morales?" He looks up, surprised. "Mr. Morales, come back in with me for a second." He obediently trots behind me back to my room.

"What happened, Mr. Morales?"

"What happened?"

"With your wife. What happened?"

He looks miserable. "We had a misunderstanding. But she called me. She said she'd be back soon."

"Did something happen to your boy?"

"No, I told her, it was an accident, nothing happened. She'll be back soon."

"Do you want to talk to someone about all this, Mr. Morales?" I feel an emergency psychiatric appointment may be in order, but he shakes his head vehemently.

"Oh, no."

"Well, at any rate, Dr. Grossman is back next week. I forgot to tell you but I know you'll be happy about that. So the next time you come in, that's two weeks from today, remember, you'll see him. OK?"

Oh, no. Mr. Morales's face is dissolving in abject misery. Devastated, he looks off into the distance. A tear rolls down his cheek.

"Mr. Morales?"

He shakes his head, unable to speak.

"Mr. Morales?"

"I can't stay with you?"

"But you missed him so much! You . . ."

He stays with me.

September 1991
March 1992

October 1992

"I know I got it in here."

Mr. Morales is rummaging through a wad of filthy papers he has extricated from a filthy shopping bag, looking for the letter he got yesterday that has sent him into a state of nervous collapse. He doesn't remember what it was about, only that he needed me to answer it urgently. I am transfixed by the sight of his fingers, filthy beyond description, stumbling clumsily through the dog-eared sheaf of official forms. Finally, he drags an envelope out from the back of the pack and hands it over.

"This is it?"

I unfold the form. It is from the Supreme Court of the State of New York and tells him that he is being called for jury duty and must reply by a date now six months in the past.

"Are you sure this is it, Mr. Morales? This is from a while ago."

He takes the letter back and scowls at it, then flips ineffectually through the packet of papers again.

"Maybe I left it at home. I got to go find it." He makes as if to head for the door and go look for it right now.

"No, no, no, don't go now. You can bring it another time, next week if you have to. Now you have to talk to me for a second."

He reluctantly settles back into the chair, still thumbing through the sheaf of papers. I have no doubt that every one of them is laden with deadlines and accumulating penalties. Should I ask to see the rest of them? I would have to put on a pair of gloves first. They are so dirty. And, formally speaking, none of my business, although as Mr. Morales begins to shimmer on my chair, increasingly vague and ineffectual, it's hard to apply the usual criteria for what is my business and what isn't. In his present state of disarray he could do with an accountant, a lawyer, a secretary, a handyman, and a wife—above all things, a wife. Instead, he has an overburdened social worker, a visiting nurse who sees him once a week, Mary, and me.

"Looks like you've been gardening!" Actually, it doesn't. There is no other polite way to broach the state of a person's fingernails.

"I'm doing some pipe work on the house."

"Plumbing?"

"Yeah. I got to get it fixed up for when she gets back."

Mary is still getting periodic phone calls from Mrs. Morales. Mrs. Morales wants to know how Mr. Morales is, how he's managing. She wants us to understand that she had no choice in doing what she did, and that she and the children are thriving. She shows no evidence of changing her mind and going back to him.

"Mr. Morales, are you sure you're OK in that house by yourself?"

The voice of his visiting nurse from the last time I talked to her echoes loud in my ears: ". . . a shambles. Indescribable."

"Oh, yes, I just got to finish a little work. She'll be back. We just had a little misunderstanding." He pauses. "Do you know where she is?"

"No, no, I don't." At least I don't have to lie about this. "Listen, Mr. Morales, have you been thinking about what we talked about last time? About moving into a place where you have people around to help you out, to cook for you . . . ?"

"I told you." He is as impatient as I've seen him get, although barely a ruffle of emotion disturbs the flat surface of his affect. "I bought the house for the kids. I want to leave it to the kids when I go. I can't move out. That neighborhood, if I go they'll tear it apart. I got to stay there. I'm doing all right."

He weighs less than a hundred pounds now, a small bundle of stained long johns, three ragged flannel shirts, a pair of woolen pants of entirely indeterminate color, and a leather jacket. And the hat, always the hat, firmly and permanently planted. It is only on rare occasions that I force him to remove two or three layers of stiff gray clothes so that I can at least approximate the stethoscope to his chest. I know without asking that he is smoking cigarettes nonstop: the brown stain on his right middle finger is visible even through the grime, and packs of Marlboros are always falling out of his shirt pockets. But other than his constant malodorous cough, he has no physical complaints. No complaints at all, for that matter. He doesn't seem to have registered his own weight loss, now about forty pounds since last year. I have supplied him with the usual appetite builders and dietary supplements, but without much enthusiasm. They won't do much for the real problem.

At Mr. Morales's last visit I left him sitting in my office and poked my head into the social worker's office to report that Mr. Morales was complaining he had no help at home. A mild and entirely justified explosion ensued:

"I got him an aide. I got him a homemaker. I got him everything, on an emergency basis. Faxes everywhere. All arranged. And he doesn't let them into the house. He has no phone, he doesn't let anyone in through the door. The agencies tried a few times, then they said forget it."

I went back to Mr. Morales. "We tried to get you help. You didn't let them in."

He was silent and looked a little confused.

"When people come to your door, do you let them in?"

"Oh, no. That neighborhood, can't let no one in."

"So how can we get you some help, if you don't let them in?"

"Yes. OK." He promised to start letting people in. Paul contacted the agencies again, and the home health aide and the homemaker got through the door the following week. But Mr. Morales fired them both a few days later: "They started stealing from me. I had to let them go. Anyway, they couldn't cook anyway." That was that.

Now the only person who gains access to the house is his visiting nurse, Maureen, who comes to him on Mondays and often calls Mary or me after her visit to decompress. During one of her first visits she toured the house with a shopping bag, collecting dozens of prescription-drug vials scattered throughout, some dating back five or ten years. This harvest would have had a more beneficial impact had she not sent the shopping bag to the clinic via Mr. Morales at his next visit. He watched me sort through the outdated amber vials, suddenly decided that he "might need" some of them someday, and firmly lugged them all back home with him again.

Maureen retaliated by making him a "pillbox," laying out his daily medications into a grid of plastic compartments so that he can take morning, noon, and night pills every day without too much thought. She reported that the compartments were indeed empty the next Monday when she returned to refill them. We all breathed a little more easily. At least a molecule of order was orbiting amidst the charged atomic chaos of Mr. Morales.

Today I can glimpse the pillbox at the bottom of the shopping bag and also, to my dismay, about a dozen suspiciously weathered amber vials. I decide to postpone an offer to look through Mr. Morales's stack of documents and concentrate on what is more clearly in my legitimate purview.

"Let's take a look at your medicines."

He obediently drags out the pillbox. It is full, every compartment of every column primed with his pills of the hour. But this is Wednesday. Why are the Monday and Tuesday columns full?

"You're not taking your medicines?"

"Yes, I'm taking them all right."

"You're supposed to be taking them from this box!"

"Oh, no."

"Oh, yes, Mr. Morales, yes. From this box."

"No, I been taking these, they're better." Out come the amber vials, one by one. Valium, prescribed by Dr. Grossman, six years old. Valium, prescribed by Dr. Grossman, four years old. Ampicillin, prescribed by me, one year old. A bottle of unidentified white pills of mixed sizes and shapes.

"I don't think she knows what she's doing, putting them in that box all mixed up," says Mr. Morales. "I didn't feel good when I was taking from the box. I like to take them from the bottles so I know what I'm getting. It's safer."

That's it for me. When I call our psychiatrist liaison on duty, I'm lucky enough to reach Dr. Ortega, who met Mr. Morales once before, years ago, during a routine evaluation for the research study, and remembers him well. She cheerfully agrees to come over to the clinic right now and formally evaluate his competence. Once he is confirmed by a psychiatrist as mentally incompetent and a danger to himself, he can be committed to a care facility, even against his will.

"Mr. Morales, do you remember Dr. Ortega?" He doesn't. "She wants to talk to you a little." He doesn't have time. Dr. Ortega, preternaturally gifted at initiating difficult interviews, somehow soothes him out to a secluded bench in the corridor. The shopping bag, exhibit A, stays with me.

An hour later Dr. Ortega returns Mr. Morales to the waiting room and pokes her head into my room.

"So?"

"I'm afraid he did pretty well."

"No. No. He's not competent. How can he be competent? Look." I fish the Valium out of the bag and shake them in her face. "He can't go back by himself with these. How can he be competent?"

She is sympathetic but firm. Conscientious psychiatrists bend over backward to avoid stripping people of their civil rights. Formally, Mr. Morales is apparently still on the "eccentric" side of the border: he understands, albeit slowly, too much of his circumstances to be legally forced anywhere for his own good. "I'll take a look at him in a few months," Dr. Ortega promises. Meanwhile, she reports, he says he needs his shopping bag back right away because he thinks he may have left the gas oven on in his kitchen. I quickly toss the vials of Valium into the trash before heading into the waiting room to hand over the shopping bag.

September 1991
March 1992
October 1992

March 1993

"Is that Dr. Zuger?"

I can't place this woman's voice on the phone. Whoever she is, I hope she will go away quickly. I have been forced to hold up an apologetic finger and stop the new patient sitting in front of me just as she has begun to haltingly describe how she lost a baby to AIDS. Why do they always put through phone calls just at the moment of tears? I try to sound unwelcoming.

"Yes."

The voice on the other end of the phone turns even more tentative. "This is Lucy Morales."

"Mrs. Morales?" For all my immersion in the Morales situation, I have never yet either seen or spoken to the wife in the safe house. Mary is her contact here.

"No. This is his daughter." His daughter? What daughter? The only daughter I know about is little, somewhere between six and ten. This voice is an adult's.

"His daughter?"

"Yes. My stepmother told me where to reach you." Ah. Stepmother. Now that she mentions it, I remember that this current marriage is Mr. Morales's second. Presumably this Lucy is issue of his first. From out of town, no doubt, but arriving not a moment too soon.

"I'm so glad to hear from you!" And if I'm glad, Maureen, Mary, and Paul will be ecstatic. "But I'll have to call you back in fifteen minutes. Where can I reach you?"

"Uh, I really have to go . . ." My sudden warmth has only made her sound even more tentative.

"No, wait, wait, let me connect you to our social worker—"

She is retreating fast. "No, really, I have to go. I just wanted to let you know that Dad is in Pelham Hospital—"

"Oh, no. What happened?"

The new patient has dried her tears and is now looking a little peeved, alternately eyeing her fingernails and me with mounting irritation. Some patients become magnanimous in their pain, but this one, I know from the set of her jaw, thinks I have rejected her tragedy in favor of someone else's. That's it for our rapport today, and possibly forever. I might as well take my time with the prodigal daughter.

"His doctor at Pelham wanted me to get in touch with you."

"But what happened?"

"He said I should get you to call him, it's Dr. Diaz, at 415-8500 beeper 824."

"OK, I'll call him. But tell me where I can reach you. Are you in town for long?"

There is a silence. "I live here."

"In the Bronx?"

"In Queens."

Ah, in Queens, safe in Queens as the flesh of her flesh, et cetera, et cetera, fades further and further from the world, barricading himself into his filthy pile of papers, pipe work, and loose planks. Last week Mary got a terse phone call from Maureen announcing that the Visiting Nurse Service had "dropped the Morales case." Maureen said that her supervisor feels Mr. Morales needs to be confined in a long-term care facility, and that continued service to the home is unnecessarily endangering the service's personnel. Maureen didn't sound too upset. Mary thinks a plank may have fallen on her. Mary called the agency to appeal this verdict, which seems unnecessarily punitive to the wrong party, but Maureen's supervisor has yet to return Mary's call. In the meantime, Mr. Morales is now entirely alone in the twilight.

"In Queens. I see." And I do. "How is he doing?"

"I don't really know," she says quickly. "I just got the call myself. He's still in the Emergency."

"I see. Well, I'll call the hospital, then. Would you like me to give you a call back?"

"No, I'm kind of hard to reach," she says. "I'll call you back."

Although she hangs up right away, I keep hold of the telephone for a moment before turning back to the stiff silence of my waiting patient in the chair.

When I page Dr. Diaz later that afternoon, I can tell from his breathlessness and the echoing clatter of the background noise that he is a young intern in a big emergency room. His initial bewilderment regarding who I am and why I'm calling leads me to hypothesize that I have caught him temporarily separated from his clipboard. The fact that I can clearly remember how frantic and helpless I used to become when separated from my list of things to ask and do, before I understood enough to ask and do them instinctively, does not make it any more fun to talk to him.

"José seems very confused," says Dr. Diaz.

José indeed.

"Mr. Morales has been confused for some time. How exactly did he get there?"

"The cops got him in off the Bronx River Parkway."

A vision of Mr. Morales walking tentatively down the divider is a terrible one, but a sudden flash of him behind the wheel of a car is even worse.

"He was walking on the Parkway?"

"He was driving on the Parkway."

Oh, Lord, the car. How could we all have forgotten about that car, completely and utterly forgotten? We haven't heard the car mentioned since Mrs. Morales stopped double-parking outside the clinic building, and just assumed she took it with her. How could we have made such a dumb mistake? How could Mr. Morales, groping tentatively through the increasingly thick mysteries of daily life, ever have retained the canniness to avoid any further mention of the car?

"Was anyone hurt?"

"Nah, he was already on the shoulder, they said. He told them he couldn't remember how to drive."

I can see two or three huge cops crouching beside the front window of an ancient Chevy while Mr. Morales, helpless as an upended tortoise behind the wheel, searches for the words to explain that he suddenly cannot remember how to get where he may or may not have been going.

On the other end of the phone, I can tell that Dr. Diaz has located his clipboard: his voice suddenly becomes brisk and businesslike. "So my resident said I should ask you, has José ever had a CT scan of his head?"

I explain the extent of the neurologic testing that has led to Mr. Morales's diagnosis of HIV encephalopathy. Dr. Diaz, although I can tell he is writing busily, is clearly unconvinced. "My resident says he needs a full neuro workup, to make sure he doesn't really have an opportunistic infection that is making him demented."

I personally know that Mr. Morales doesn't need a full new workup, my experience with demented HIV-infected patients exceeding the combined total of that of

Dr. Diaz and his resident by a factor of ten, but I'm not about to say so. What Mr. Morales needs is anything that will keep him safe out of his house and off the streets, safe in a facility where someone will take care of him and arrange for his further care. If a few unnecessary tests and procedures are the price of this respite, then so be it.

"That sounds fine. But listen, Dr. Diaz, you must absolutely not let him go home when this workup is over, OK?"

"Not go home?"

"He needs placement in some kind of nursing home. He absolutely cannot go back to his own house." I fill Dr. Diaz in on the Morales homestead, but although he listens politely, the reassurances I long to hear, that the long and solitary Morales odyssey is over, are not forthcoming. Dr. Diaz is silent.

"You see, don't you? That he can't go back there?"

"His daughter already told me, she doesn't want him in a nursing home."

"Yeah, listen, where did you find this daughter?"

"José said to call her. He had her number in his wallet."

Wait till I tell Paul that Mr. Morales has been hoarding a potential custodian who could have solved all our problems a long time ago. On the other hand, my brief contact with the daughter didn't augur well for that kind of help from her.

"Look, this daughter hasn't really been involved with his care at all. I'm not sure you should pay a great deal of attention to what she says."

Dr. Diaz may not have been a doctor for very long, but it has been long enough for him to have learned a few basics. He clearly knows, for instance, how much easier it is to send a patient home from the hospital than to try to arrange direct admission to a nursing home, where endless forms, endless lines, and strict admission criteria stymie most transfers for weeks or months.

"We would really prefer if possible to send José home."

José. My God, he has known Mr. Morales for about four and a half hours and is now controlling his destiny and some of my own as well. But this is, of course, how the system works. I have no authority over Dr. Diaz, his resident, or Pelham Hospital. All I can do is try to explain to them how things have been, and hope someone exercises some sense in determining how things will be.

A beeper sounds loudly into the phone.

"I have to go," says Dr. Diaz.

"All right, look, please keep me posted, OK?"

"You bet, " says Dr. Diaz, mightily relieved that this conversation is now drawing to a close. "His daughter says she's coming in to see him tonight, so we'll talk to her again about a nursing home. His wife is coming too.

"His wife? I don't think . . ."

"José says his wife will come too."

September 1991
March 1992
October 1992
March 1993

September 1993

Mr. Morales, his wife, and his home health aide are crowded into my examining room on chairs I have lugged in from the waiting room. Each one looks more uncomfortable than the next. The aide, a tall, asthenic young man in blue jeans and earrings, reaches around to help Mr. Morales take off his coat. Mrs. Morales, plump and middle-aged, also in blue jeans and earrings, is already helping him off with his coat. They tangle briefly behind the oblivious back of Mr. Morales, who is looking off into the distance as his toothpick arms are jerked slightly from side to side.

"I got it."

"No, I got it."

They subside, then look up at me expectantly. Mr. Morales looks at his lap. I feel completely unequal to the next half hour.

Against all odds, Mrs. Morales did make a beeline straight from her safe house to Pelham Hospital six months ago, drawn by who knows how many tautening cords of guilt, sentiment, obligation, and curiosity. A tearful reunion among husband, wife, and stepdaughter evidently took place over Mr. Morales's hospital bed. All reaffirmed their determination that Mr. Morales would live out his life in his own home, with his own family nearby. His grown daughter, Lucy, immediately headed over to the house to fix and tidy what she could. Contact with the Visiting Nurse Service was reestablished. A representative of the agency toured the house after Lucy's ministrations and deemed it no longer a risk to their nurses. The agency agreed to reopen the Morales case, with the provision that this time a member of the family would be available for backup. The VNS often insists on backup—a family member or other responsible party nearby—for difficult cases, just in case things get out of hand. If no backup can be located, no nursing service is provided— "Too risky for our personnel." Of course, the patients with no possible backup are exactly the ones that need nursing services the most, but pointing this out to the agency is, we have learned, a futile exercise in abstract reasoning.

Lucy, off in Queens, lived too far away to be an acceptable backup. A sister of Mr. Morales's unearthed in Co-op City was uninterested in getting involved. No one was left but Mrs. Morales, still living in her safe house for battered wives and children, which, she divulged for the first time, was an hour and a half north of the city, deep in the Westchester suburbs. There she and her two small children shared a pleasant room. The kids had enrolled in the local public schools. Was Mrs. Morales about to uproot them yet again, to haul them back to the innards of the inner city, to a house even more dilapidated than it was two years ago, to grimy, dangerous schools, to a father who, although not perhaps formally a batterer in the literal sense of the word, was far from ideal in most respects?

She was not, she explained stolidly over and over again to Dr. Diaz, to his supervisors, to an endless stream of social workers at Pelham Hospital. Those kids were going to stay right where they were. She herself was prepared to put herself out for her husband to whatever lengths were deemed necessary, but surely they could see that the children were best left out of the backup loop.

And so we have come to the present arrangement. Mrs. Morales and her children continue to live in a safe house for battered women and children, some ninety minutes north of the city, in an undisclosed location, with an unlisted phone number. Mrs. Morales has informed the administration of the safe house that she has been lucky enough to find a live-in housekeeping job Monday through Friday in the city. She spends Monday through Friday living with Mr. Morales and a rotation of around-the-clock health aides in his home in the middle of the Bronx. Maureen comes by to visit every Monday, as before. Through Maureen, Mrs. Morales has informed the Visiting Nurse Service of a weekend housekeeping job she has been lucky enough to find in the suburbs. She packs up and departs for it every Friday evening. A next-door neighbor of Mr. Morales, an elderly woman with her own array of twenty-four-hour home help, has agreed to serve as Mr. Morales's weekend backup, while Mrs. Morales is out of town, at an undisclosed location, with an undisclosed phone number, with the undisclosed children she purportedly sent to their grandmother in Puerto Rico months ago.

Contrary to all sane predictions, they are all now in their fifth month of this whirligig. Of them all, Mr. Morales, now barely conscious of his surroundings, seems to be making out the best. He does very little now but sit by the window of his house and smoke, through the days and through the nights. Sometimes he coughs. He rarely speaks, and has apparently foresworn eating and sleeping completely. Around him, the still center of the household, Mrs. Morales and the aides buzz in constant activity. Every couple of weeks they reenact it all in my examining room.

"He still doesn't sleep," says Mrs. Morales now. "He needs something for sleep."

"And to eat," says the aide. "He needs that Marinol for the appetite." The aide has a extensive knowledge of HIV therapeutics, gleaned either through prior nursing assignments or through his own prescriptions, I'm not sure which. Many of his suggestions would be right on the mark were Mr. Morales not perched so clearly on the verge of another world.

"Last night he kept telling me to turn the lights on," says Mrs. Morales. "I tell him over and over that they're on, but he doesn't listen. Then he sends me out to get light bulbs. I tell him we already got the brightest, but no, I got to go out and get more."

"He needs testosterone shots," the aide says.

"He's coughing all the time."

"I don't like his color. He needs EPO shots."

"He don't sleep, is the real problem. No more than fifteen minutes at a time."

"Maureen gave me this for you." The aide hands over a brief note from Maureen, telling me that Mr. Morales is coughing green phlegm and running a low-grade temperature and that she needs me to fill out Medicaid forms for a hospital bed, a shower seat, and a walker.

"He needs an antibiotic," the aide says. "Definitely. He needs Cipro."

"No, that Cipro gave him the rash," says Mrs. Morales.

"That was fungus, that rash."

"That was the Cipro, that's why we stopped giving it, remember, the rash came and we stopped giving it?"

"The rash was from fungus."

"It was from Cipro, he got real sick with that pill."

The aide purses his lips and shakes his head. Mrs. Morales turns back to me.

"He needs something stronger to sleep."

I used to play an active role in these discussions. Now I tend to sit them out. I let the bickering run on while I gaze at Mr. Morales, wizened and crumpled as a dried mushroom, swathed in sweaters, leather cap wobbling loosely over his ears.

"Mr. Morales?"

He looks at me hesitantly, says nothing.

"How are you, Mr. Morales?"

He looks a little like he is about to tell me, but nothing comes out.

"Can I listen to your chest?"

I try to insinuate the stethoscope behind his shoulder blades, but too many sweaters intervene.

"Can I help you up on the table here?" He offers no objection.

Mrs. Morales and the aide move slightly out of the way as I hoist Mr. Morales into a standing position and try to wiggle him over to the table. Mrs. Morales reaches out to help, but neither of us is very strong.

"Let the man do it," Mr. Morales says suddenly. His voice is cracked and rusty. "It's not that I don't think you're strong enough, but he's a man. I feel more comfortable with him."

Mrs. Morales shrugs and moves out of the way into the corner of the room, her face falling. I transfer the dead weight to the aide, who competently hoists Mr. Morales up onto the table and stays by him, one arm balancing him by the shoulders with a delicate touch, the other reaching over quickly to realign the cap to a rakish angle over the knobby scalp.

"He's doing very well," the aide says. "He's doing excellent. Aren't you, José?"

"Excellent," Mrs. Morales echoes from the corner.

Nancy Corelli

JUNE 1993

Nancy is sitting in the waiting room bent over a magazine, half an hour early for her appointment and looking fine. Year after year now, as the others out there slowly fade into shadows, she has remained solid, substantial, voluptuous, the only image left on the screen.

She first came to our clinic about five years ago for an HIV test. It was her fifth. The others had all been positive, but Nancy, refusing to believe the unbelievable, still felt there was the possibility of a mistake and had no patience for anyone who suggested otherwise.

"I don't trust any doctor but Dr. Brandon," she announced, standing in the middle of my examining room and looking belligerent. She was referring to the doctor in our group who had cared for Michael, her second husband and passport to infection, during his final days.

The temptation in these situations is always to usher the disappointed party directly into the office of the beloved, but Dr. Brandon's clinic attendance was irregular, and that busy afternoon his cubicle was dark. Nancy glowered at this news, shrugged, cracked her gum, and sat. We had clearly made each other's day.

She was all show. Despite the lush classical profile taken directly from a Roman coin, despite the deep voice, the bright golden hair, the stretch denim jeans and punishing heels, despite her early departure from all forms of organized education, Nancy proved to have all the charm and savvy of an orphaned pup. By her second visit (the test was positive) she was giving me details of her love life. When Dr. Brandon reappeared a month later, she was unmoved. She belonged to me.

At the beginning I didn't suspect what I was getting into. Technically speaking, in the spectrum of the HIV-infected, Nancy was, and still is, asymptomatic. The virus, latent in her body, is causing no medical problems at all.

Her immune system is still working. Technically speaking, all Nancy would be needing from me in the clinic was a wave and a wink from time to time.

In fact, for the first few years of our acquaintance, she was almost a full-time job. She had aches and twinges, numbness and tingling, rashes and wheezes, terrible breathlessness, and a continual rippling of her sight. Her symptoms always came on at night, in the dark. I could never find anything wrong.

Finally I caught on. Michael had died blind, numb, and screaming, and Nancy knew all too well what to expect for herself. "Just tell me how long," she would plead. "Just say, 'More than five years,' or 'Less than five years.' Just tell me when."

It took a long time to get her to believe that if I could have told her, I would have. Instead of a prognosis Nancy has had to settle for statistics, and at this point the statistics are not very helpful in predicting futures like hers.

The great majority of people in Nancy's situation have gone on to develop severe immunocompromise or AIDS after a grace period that ranges from a few years to more than a dozen. A small, baffling minority have remained absolutely well, living with the virus with no apparent ill effects. AZT given at the right time seems able to prolong the grace period for some people, but not for all. The chances are that other prophylactic regimens more successful than AZT will come off the drawing board at some point in the near future. No one can predict quite when.

Meanwhile, they all ask us the same questions; we tell them all the same things. "Probably, but not definitely." "Nobody can predict exactly when." "Things will be changing over the next few years." They nod, shrug, smile, go home to husbands and wives, to friends, to children, to empty rooms. How do they live? That answer is never in our clinic rooms, never in our charts.

It's not in Nancy's medical record, which, despite the false alarms, the frantic phone calls, the emergency visits, is as bland as they come. Nothing has happened to her. Her vision is fine. No blotches or bumps have ever been located by me. Her blood tests are normal. Her cholesterol's a little high. Nobody looking into that chart would have a clue to the HIV-infected Nancy who unfolded in my clinic room.

When we first met she had a life composed mostly of souvenirs. Her first husband had died years ago, leaving her with Danny, now twelve. From Michael, her second husband, she got her infection and the vivid nightmare of his passing. Raymond, the third and possibly worst bargain of them all, drank, used drugs, and slugged her periodically as a record of his possession.

At some point after that fifth (and last) HIV test, Nancy managed to reset the balance of power. None of us can imagine how or why—and none of us has worked up the nerve to ask her. My own theory is that she simply had to demonstrate what an outrageous error in bookkeeping somebody had made in sending her a comeuppance clearly intended for someone else.

It was quite a show. Month after month, Nancy came into the clinic with new reports.

She got her high school equivalency diploma. ("Do you think I could become a nurse?")

She got Raymond out of her house and life. ("I miss him but, it's like, when he says he's going to be different I don't believe him.")

She got Danny through elementary school on the honor roll. ("Do you think I should tell him why we come to this clinic all the time?")

Slowly, she got rid of her symptoms. ("I knew you would say it was nothing, so when I looked again it wasn't there.")

And now she's gotten herself out of the South Bronx. ("I'm so scared I can't sleep.") She borrowed money to buy a plot of land and a mobile home in North Carolina, in the community where Danny's grandparents live. She's packed up her apartment and reserved a twenty-foot truck. They're leaving an hour after Danny graduates from sixth grade.

Tomorrow Nancy's psychiatrist from the clinic, the Legal Aid lawyer who drafted her will, and I are going to take her out to a good-bye lunch. This is something we don't ordinarily do. Our good-byes are generally said at the bedside, rarely scheduled in advance over tuna.

I suppose it should be a cheerful occasion—after all, how many graduations from our clinic, or from life with a Raymond, or from the South Bronx, do we get to celebrate? But what I realize now, as Nancy looks up from her magazine in the waiting room and waves at me, is that all I want is for her to stay with us ("How long, Dr. Zuger? Just tell me how long. Can't you just say, 'Probably never'? Can't you say it just for me?") until I can tell her everything she wants to hear.

Epilogue

Deborah Sweet lost consciousness in her aunt's house about eight weeks after her stroke. Her aunt, sobbing, had her rushed to the emergency room, where she died despite all efforts at resuscitation.

Michael Soto had a biopsy showing that the mass in his brain was the untreatable malignant lymphoma we had feared. He received radiation to the tumor and medicines to minimize swelling of the brain, but his speech never returned and his alertness faded. About ten days after the biopsy he became short of breath, and signs of worsening pneumonia developed on his chest X ray. He died in the hospital a few days later. Mrs. Soto and Melissa returned to Puerto Rico to live with her family there.

Cynthia Wilson stayed physically well for several months but her relationship with her daughters deteriorated, and both of them ultimately left her to live in group homes. Cynthia hated her empty apartment and stayed more and more with her mother. On Christmas Day 1993 Pauline Wilson's asthma suddenly started to act up. Cynthia called an ambulance, but Pauline died of asthma before the ambulance got to the hospital. The children in Pauline's care were placed in foster homes. Cynthia became depressed, weak, and confused. She signed herself into a nursing home and stopped coming to our clinic.

Lydia Rios died in her sleep. Eddie struggled alone with the children, resisting all well-meaning efforts on the part of relatives and various social service agencies to place them elsewhere. During his once- or twice-weekly visits to the clinic we noticed that his exuberance was becoming a little wilder and less logical. He began to have trouble with his memory and with the use of his legs. Nikki was soon pushing him to the clinic in her mother's old wheelchair. Eddie was briefly admitted to the hospital, where tests showed that he had developed a degeneration of the brain and spinal cord caused by HIV. He was sent to a nursing home, signed himself out after less than eight hours, and returned home, where he found that his children had been removed by relatives. He stayed alone in the apartment for a few days, until the police took him to another hospital in the South Bronx. I don't know what happened to him or his children.

Anita Lewis was admitted to the intensive care unit with a severe case of recurrent PCP. She did well. Ten days after she was admitted, as I was sitting in my cubicle in the clinic, my door opened and there she was, in a satin bathrobe and fuzzy slippers. She had come to say hello (and thank you). She signed out of the hospital shortly thereafter, without completing her treatment. I never saw her again.

Shannon never came back to the clinic for the results of her HIV test. Still, when the social worker with whom she had formed a deep and affectionate bond telephoned, Shannon did agree to a meeting. The social worker told her that her HIV test was negative. Shannon reacted with fury, announcing that she was going to sue us all for "treating her like she had AIDS." Then she disappeared for good. Even Jack didn't know where she was. A few months later our social worker got a call from the police, who had found Shannon dead of a heroin overdose in an apartment in Manhattan. In her wallet were our social worker's business card and the clinic card for another AIDS clinic in the city. A sticker listing her appointments on the back of the card indicated that she was being seen there biweekly.

Mrs. Morales loaded Mr. Morales into the car one day and drove him to Pelham Hospital, where she left him in the emergency room "for his cough." The staff at Pelham was unable to get in touch with her after that. Mr. Morales died soon after, on the Pelham wards.

Nancy is fine. She is thinking of enrolling in a nursing course in North Carolina and writes to me from time to time.

The clinic was remodeled and expanded. Each examining room now has a sink.

After Mr. Soto died I took a brief vacation from the clinic. I missed him very much. It was beginning to seem that wherever I turned ghosts were at my elbow, gaunt faces and bodies I knew as well as my own. I couldn't see a new patient without the old ones crowding in. But after a few months away from the clinic the serenity became very empty. I am now back at work.

July 1995
New York City

Acknowledgments

This book may leave readers with the illusion that medical care for a person with AIDS consists of doctor and patient facing each other across a desk, month after month, year after year, a world of therapeutics entire within a tiny cubicle. Nothing could be further from the truth. The world of medical care extends far outside the closed door to that cubicle. What goes on within is only one piece of the process.

The stories I have told, factual in all other respects, are stylized into fiction by this one: that my coworkers in the clinic remain out of focus throughout, shadows on the horizon. I must trust in the reader's good sense to understand the deeply collaborative nature of the process of medical care and to realize that it only intensifies when the disease is AIDS, when the patients are our patients, and the hospital our hospital.

I would like to offer my thanks to each one of my colleagues, who, caring for these patients and others like them, have made this book possible:

Receptionists Cheryl Farrington, Kevin Lebby, Lisa Perez;

Nutritionists Liesbeth Fernandez, Cleo Tanedo;

Social Workers Pablo Burgos, Marcia Caesar, Monnie Callan, Joe Flanagan, Liz Hurwitz;

Nurses Hazel Clayton, Jean Dugan, Amelia Hughes, Pat Kahl, Pat Klass, Barbara McKenzie, Heidi Wondra;

Physician's Assistant Cathy Pollard;

Nurse-practitioner Margaret Coffey;

Doctors Kemper Alston, Enrico Belgrave, Tom Birch, Michael Crooks, Jane Eason, Marcia Epstein, Jerry Friedland, John Froude, Larry Hanau, Kathleen Hanley, Rick Hecht, Bob Klein, Simon Liederman, Frank Lowy, Mary Alice O'Dowd, Maria Pitaro, Lew Schrager, Jon Shuter, Neal Steigbigel, David Tompkins, Barry Zingman.

To my editor, Elizabeth Knoll, I owe thanks for many years of enthusiasm and support. To Nancy Brooks and Mary Louise Byrd at W. H. Freeman and Company I offer a salute for their deft midwifery of manuscript to book.

To Michael Simberkoff, M.D., Professor of Medicine and Infectious Diseases, still hard at work in the AIDS clinic where he trained me almost a decade ago, I owe a particular debt of gratitude for his enduring example as teacher, scholar, and clinician and for many personal and professional kindnesses.

Finally, to Kathleen McCarthy, R.N., and Loretta Sullivan, F.N.P., more than thanks are due. Kathy and Loretta were the backbone, the energy, the life, and the conscience of the clinic described in these pages. They will recognize some of their old friends here, and they should know that, though not in this book themselves, during its creation they were never far from my heart.